Recent Results in Cancer Research

Fortschritte der Krebsforschung

Progrès dans les recherches sur le cancer

42

Breast Cancer:

A Challenging Problem

Edited by

M. L. Griem · E. V. Jensen · J. E. Ultmann · R. W. Wissler

With 60 Figures

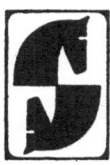

Springer-Verlag Berlin Heidelberg GmbH 1973

Symposium on Breast Cancer: A Challenging Problem
The University of Chicago Pritzker School of Medicine, March 4th and 5th, 1972

Sponsored by the Swiss League against Cancer

ISBN 978-3-642-85834-5   ISBN 978-3-642-85832-1 (eBook)
DOI 10.1007/978-3-642-85832-1

Preface

This volume summarizes the proceedings of the fifth biennial Cancer Teaching Symposium held on March 4 and 5, 1972 at the University of Chicago Pritzker School of Medicine. The program was prepared by Drs. MELVIN GRIEM, ELWOOD JENSEN, HAROLD SUTTON, JOHN ULTMANN, and ROBERT WISSLER. The purpose of the symposium was to present the current status of the challenging cancer problem, breast carcinoma, to the staff and students of this medical center and to students and interested physicians from other institutions in the Chicago area. In a fashion similar to the other teaching symposia held in 1964, 1966, 1968, and 1970, this symposium attracted over 450 physicians and scientists. In the course of one and one half days the audience had the opportunity to listen to 18 invited speakers and to the lively discussions. The formal presentations are recorded in these pages.

This teaching symposium could not have been undertaken without the faithful assistance of the program committee, the cancer training grant education committee, the staff who recorded and transcribed the proceedings, and the editorial assistants. We wish to thank the following for their efforts: JULIE KANT, Administrative Secretary for the Clinical Cancer Training Grant, as well as Dr. JAMES MARKS, MARGARET WOEHRLE, FRIEDA RANNEY, and ROSIE BARTLETT.

This symposium received financial support from USPHS Clinical Cancer Training Grant 5T12 CA-08077-06 and from the Chicago Tumor Institute.

MELVIN L. GRIEM, M. D.
ROBERT W. WISSLER, Ph. D., M. D.

Contents

List of Participants

N. I. BERLIN, Breast Cancer Task Force, National Cancer Institute, National Institutes of Health, Bethesda, MD

W. J. BURDETTE, Department of Surgery, M. D. Anderson Hospital and Tumor Institute, Houston, TX

P. P. CARBONE, Medicine Branch, National Cancer Institute, National Institutes of Health, Bethesda, MD

T. L. DAO, Department of Breast Surgery and Endocrine Research Laboratory, Roswell Park Memorial Institute, Buffalo, NY

R. L. EGAN, Department of Radiology, Emory University School of Medicine, Atlanta, GA

M. L. GRIEM, Department of Radiology, University of Chicago, Chicago, IL

G. A. HEPPNER, Division of Bio-Medical Science, Brown University, Providence, RI

L. O. JACOBSON, Division of Biological Sciences, University of Chicago, Chicago, IL

E. V. JENSEN, Ben May Laboratory, University of Chicago, Chicago, IL

R. M. KELLEY, Department of Medicine, Harvard Medical School, Boston, MA

B. J. KENNEDY, Department of Medicine, University of Minnesota School of Medicine, Minneapolis, MN

A. H. LETTON, Emory University, Atlanta, GA; American Cancer Society, Inc., New York, NY

M. B. LIPSETT, National Institute of Child Health and Human Development, National Institutes of Health, Bethesda, MD

M. L. MENDELSOHN, Department of Radiology, University of Pennsylvania, Philadelphia, PA

M. H. MYERS, End Results Group, National Cancer Institute, National Institutes of Health, Bethesda, MD

R. NISSEN-MEYER, Medical Department, Aker Hospital, Oslo, Norway

W. D. RIDER, Ontario Cancer Institute, Toronto, Canada

N. H. SARKAR, Institute for Medical Research, Camden, NJ

D. G. SCARPELLI, Department of Pathology, University of Kansas Medical Center, Kansas City, KS

M. B. SHIMKIN, Department of Community Medicine, School of Medicine, University of California at San Diego, La Jolla, CA

J. E. ULTMANN, Department of Medicine, University of Chicago, Chicago, IL

R. W. WISSLER, Department of Pathology, University of Chicago, Chicago, IL

Introduction

The Cancer Education Committee selected the topic, breast cancer, because it represents a perplexing problem as well as a very important one. We wished to present to the students the difficulties and the challenges associated with attemps to improve prevention, diagnosis and especially treatment of this common neoplasm that leads to so much suffering and death.

The real challenge and magnitude of the problem was set forth by Dr. LETTON in his opening remarks. His initial presentation laid the foundation upon which the subsequent one and one-half days were built.

Dr. SHIMKIN presented the epidemiology of breast cancer as it is understood today. Knowledge of possible causative factors, particularly viruses, hormonal factors and other agents that might increase the frequency of breast cancer, were reviewed by Dr. SARKAR and Dr. LIPSETT.

Dr. KENNEDY discussed the nature of breast cancer as it is seen in the patient; the presenting symptoms, the methods of spread, and the natural progression of the disease.

Improved methods of diagnosis were discussed by Dr. EGAN. This was followed by new evidence concerning the histological, histochemical and ultrastructural aspects of this disease, presented by Dr. SCARPELLI. Dr. JENSEN described criteria for predicting which patients are responsive to endocrine therapy, and Dr. HEPPNER outlined immunological management of breast cancer. The dynamics of breast cancer growth in relation to cell kinetics and the possible implications of this knowledge were discussed by Dr. MENDELSOHN.

The current status of treatment of breast cancer was reviewed by Dr. MYERS, who surveyed the end results of treatment and outlined the problem of the late recurrence of this disease following apparently successful initial therapy. Dr. RIDER, Dr. BURDETTE and Dr. NISSEN-MEYER reviewed the current methods of approaching the patient with a primary lesion in the breast, discussing various surgical, radiotherapeutic, hormonal, and chemotherapeutic approaches to the management of breast cancer.

Metastatic breast cancer and its management were discussed by Dr. DAO and Dr. KELLEY. An excellent summary of the symposium was given by Dr. CARBONE.

The editors are grateful to all the participants who worked so hard to make this teaching symposium a success and to bring this monograph to fruition.

M. L. GRIEM, E. V. JENSEN,
J. E. ULTMANN, R. W. WISSLER

Opening of the Symposium

March 4 and 5, 1972

L. O. JACOBSON

It is in a sense a coincidence that this teaching symposium is being held at this time when so much new attention and new support is being given to solve this very important health problem—the problem of breast cancer. We are fortunate indeed to have so many of the national and international leaders in the field here to share their knowledge and the results of their labors with us. It is fascinating to me in just looking at the program to see the enormous progress that has been made in the understanding of breast cancer in the past 20 years or so. It's true that it hasn't gone as rapidly as many of you think it should; but I believe that in the last 5 years the momentum, the interest and the interaction among scientists, teachers, and clinicians has increased to the point that progress is likely to be very swift indeed in the next decade. We are especially pleased to have all of you here for this next day and a half. I welcome you not only as the Dean of the Division and the Medical School but on behalf of the University as well. I know that each of the audience here will gain much from the presentations, and I'm convinced that even the participants will learn something from each other. I wish you well.

The Challenge of Cancer of the Breast

A. Hamblin Letton

The magnitude of the breast cancer problem is much greater than is generally realized. It is the number one killer of women in the United States. There are roughly 70,000 new cases each year, with 31,000 deaths each year from cancer of the breast. These figures are hard for us to realize unless we translate them into the experiences of our every day life. The new cases of breast cancer each year would fill Yankee Stadium with standing room only—more women develop breast cancer than the total automobile accident deaths in the United States each year—in ten years the incidence of breast cancer exceeds the population of Boston, Massachusetts—in the ten years of the Vietnam War, 310,000 women have died from cancer of the breast, while we have lost 36,920 servicemen in East Asia. One out of every fifteen newborn girls will develop cancer of the breast. In every seventeen minute period, three new cases of breast cancer will be diagnosed and in those same seventeen minutes, one woman will die of cancer of the breast. The mortality rate of cancer of the breast has remained very nearly 25 per 100,000 over the past forty years.

Does this mean that we are not improving our cure rate during this period of time? No! It is coincidental that the incident rate has increased the same as the cure rate has increased. In Connecticut [1] where the State Registry has been active for a number of years, the incident rate has increased from 55 per 100,000 in 1940—44, to 72 per 100,000 in 1965—68, which means that we are curing almost 20% more women now than we were curing thirty years ago. This is due, in the main, to earlier detection, for the treatment for this malady has experienced very little change in this period of time. Collected statistics [2] show that only 45% of patients with cancer of the breast who have positive axillary nodes are being cured, while 85% can be cured when there is no nodal involvement. Statistics therefore show that through the educational efforts, mainly of the American Cancer Society, we are treating breast cancer earlier today than ever before. Our efforts are paying off, but not enough. How can this be improved? How can the mortality rate of cancer of the breast be further reduced? Simply stated, the problem apparently is not so much in improving our methods of therapy, for we have proved that we can cure early cancer of the breast—our problem is how to find more breast cancers earlier. The modalities which we have at present to find more cancers earlier are, first, public education—increasing the number of women practicing breast self-examination and annual examinations. Second, professional education—causing our physicians to suspect cancer more often—to utilize consultations with cancer oriented physicians earlier—to use proper diagnostic aids. The American Cancer Society has been advocating these modalities through the years, but we must renew and increase our efforts to convince more women to do breast self-examination and get annual checkups. We must convince more physicians to suspect cancer more often—to examine the patient more carefully—to utilize mammography and thermography to better advantage.

I have been very impressed by the reports of GILBERTSON [3] at the Cancer Detection Center at the University of Minnesota, where some 8,000 women, 45 years or older, have undergone 46,000 annual examinations. For those in which cancer of the breast was found, this has resulted in an observed survival rate of 96%, 86% and 82% at the five, ten and fifteen year intervals, which is a relative survival rate of 104%, 105% und 119% at these same intervals. It dramatically shows that early cancer of the breast can be detected by annual physical examination.

The work by MARTIN and GALLAGER [4] of Houston, Texas, is also impressive. They report that they are able to diagnose *in situ* cancer of the breast by the appearance of a new density in serial mammograms. *In situ* cancer of the breast should be 100% curable.

The mass screening techniques of PHILLIP STRAX [5] of the Guttmann Institute in New York City where, with a combination of mammography, thermography and clinical examination, he reports only missing two cancers out of 9,000 consecutive examinations. His ability to find early lesions, at the time of the subsequent examination, is another example of how annual screening examinations are of great value in reducing this mortality rate.

The hope of reducing the mortality rate in the future lies in some combination of these techniques.

The Board of Directors of the American Cancer Society, at their February 1972 meeting, approved a proposal and guidelines for launching a major program of earlier detection of breast cancer, including the following approaches:

1. Expansion of the Public Education Program of breast self-examination.

2. Expansion of the Professional Education Program to alert physicians to the importance of earlier diagnosis and to inform them about adequate clinical examination plus the effectiveness of radiologic techniques and thermography.

3. Encouragement of periodic clinical breast examination.

4. Providing support for the training of personnel and the development of new facilities and/or the enlargement of existing breast cancer facilities, as demonstration projects.

5. Providing support for the clinical investigation projects which evaluate newer modalities of promise in the field of early diagnosis.

The goals of this program are the discovery of breast cancer at a stage most amenable to cure, therefore, to reduce the mortality rate further. At that time, the Board also allocated $ 2 million to initiate this program.

The Cancer Act of 1971 causes the American Cancer Society to accept a greater responsibility than ever before. The Research Department is preparing to increase its activities. It is, even now, receiving an increased number of requests for research grants and requests for training research personnel—also, it must serve as a second source for cancer research funds. It is not wise to allow a monopoly to occur in support of any research project and it is particularly important that we should not let the National Cancer Institute furnish all of the funding for cancer research. One of the distinctive features of the Research Program of the American Cancer Society, and a most important one, is the input by dedicated laymen, as well as knowledgeable scientists and physicians. Therefore, our research effort must be expanded.

When the results of the renewed and enlarged research effort starts giving us new ways to diagnose and treat cancer, the American Cancer Society is going to have a greater responsibility than ever before—a responsibility to keep the public informed— that they may know where to go and seek this new help at the proper time. We must also keep the physician informed—that they may know how and when to apply the new methods of diagnosis and treatment, so more and more patients can be cured.

The American Cancer Society will also find an increasing demand for the Service and Rehabilitation Programs. These programs include those which rehabilitate the colostomy, laryngectomy, amputee and the mastectomy patients. Programs which will help with transportation, with lending sick room equipment, with drugs for pain and with chemotherapy. I would dare say that our program here today and tomorrow will result in more women being successfully treated for cancer of the breast which will cause a greater need for the mastectomy rehabilitation services.

We must acknowledge that, at the present time, we are unable to prevent cancer of the breast, but that we can cure it and we are curing it in increasing numbers. What of those that we do cure? How many of the 39,000 victims of cancer of the breast, which we will cure this year, will learn that their ability to find life satisfying has been impaired? How many will find quality of survival? In St. Matthews it is written, "what does it profiteth a man if he gains the whole world and loses his soul", you might paraphrase this to say, "what does it profiteth the woman to cure her of cancer of the breast and she loses her ability to live a full life". If you remove her breast, how will she respond socially—how will her family react—will her husband meet this new challenge—will her children—will her associates? This is the importance of the rehabilitation of breast cancer patients and their families. I recently met a charming woman in Florida, whose husband divorced her immediately after her mastectomy. What did it profit her to cure her of cancer of the breast? She was despondent and felt she was a social outcast, not only by her husband but by her associates. She felt rejected. The American Cancer Society's Reach to Recovery Program found her and made it possible for her to be able to communicate with other women who had had mastectomy and who had overcome these difficulties. Through this experience and in the printed word of the American Cancer Society's Reach to Recovery literature, she learned how to react, how to dress and how to face life again. She is now a vibrant and enthusiastic citizen, meeting her obligations to her children and to society.

I notice that there is nothing in this program concerning the rehabilitation of the breast cancer patient and, therefore, let me stress to you how strongly I feel that we have a responsibility to our patients which does not end when the wound is healed, but we must extend our concern for our patients the rest of the way to total physical and social recovery and rehabilitation, that our patients may find quality of survival.

Let me congratulate you on the excellent program which I see coming in the next few hours, today and tomorrow, and congratulate you on pinpointing your attention to this Number One killer and crippler of women. I think that things learned and things said here today can help to save the lives of countless women.

References

1. CUTLER, S. J., CHRISTINE, B., BARCLAY, T. H. C.: Increasing Incidents and Decreasing Mortality Rates for Breast Cancer. Cancer (Philad.) 28, 1376—1380 (1971).
2. Facts and Figures. American Cancer Society, 1971.
3. GILBERTSON, V. A., KJELSBURG, M.: Detection of Breast Cancer by Periodic Utilization Methods of Physical Diagnosis. Cancer (Philad.) 28, 1552—1554 (1971).
4. MARTIN, J. E., GALLAGER, H. S.: Mammographic Diagnosis of Minimal Cancer. Cancer (Philad.) 28, 1519—1526 (1971).
5. STRAX, P.: Personal Presentation to the Task Force on Breast Cancer. American Cancer Society, 1971.

Epidemiology of Breast Cancer

M. B. Shimkin

Cancer of the mammary gland is one of the more common neoplasms among several mammalian species, including man, dog, rat and mouse.

Cancer of the breast in man is one of the earliest neoplasms to be described in medical writings. It has been used as the model for many generalizations about neoplasms since the days of Hippocrates. And laboratory cancer research practically started with mammary tumours in mice [18].

Distribution

The World Health Organization [7] has collected incidence rates of cancer in over 40 areas on 5 continents, to add to the older cancer mortality statistics such as compiled by Segi [25].

Table 1 extracts the incidence rates in 8 localities around the world, illustrating the extremes. The highest rates are in the United States, among the so-called white

Table 1. Annual incidence rates for breast cancer per 100,000 females, age-standardized to a world population [7]

High	Rate/100,000
U.S.A. (white)	62.3—62.4
U.K.	42.5—51.1
Scandinavia	41.0—48.6
Intermediate	
Cali, Colombia	27.3
Yugoslavia	22.8
Bombay, India	20.4
Low	
South Africa (black)	11.9—13.6
Japan	11.0—12.4

populations of Connecticut and Alameda County, California. The lowest rates are in Japan and the black population of South Africa. Intermediate rates include sites in Europe, South America and Asia, the latter being Bombay.

The difference between the highest and the lowest rates is approximately 6 to 1. In cancer sites with important known environmental determinants, such as the uterine cervix and the esophagus, the extremes are 15 and over 100 to 1, respectively.

Breast cancer occurs only rarely in males, the usual ratio being approximately 1 male to 100 females.

Breast cancer incidence increases with age, but the slope of the curve becomes flatter at older age groups, with the "break" at the age of menopause. Fig. 1, taken from DE WAARD [6] demonstrates this feature. It is not clear whether this change in slope indicates that there are two different diseases in the present rubric for breast cancer or whether this is an effect of hormonal or other changes with age in the host. My prejudices favor the latter explanation.

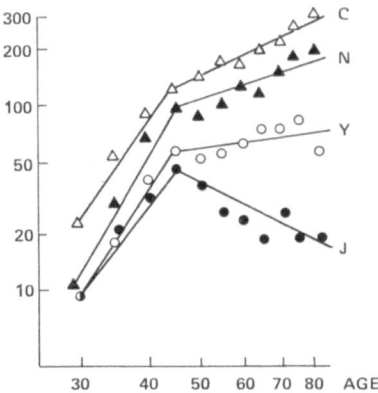

Fig. 1. Age-specific incidence of breast cancer plotted on a logarithmic scale, showing the "break" at the menopausal age, for Connecticut (C), Norway (N), Yugoslavia (Y) and Japan (J). From DE WAARD [6]

Several authors [14, 29] have commented upon the steady-state of breast cancer morbidity and mortality in the United States during the past 30 or more years. Incidence data from Connecticut [5] recently demonstrated increases among younger women, although the mortality rate was not affected. The 1969 third survey of cancer morbidity [2] in the United States shows an annual sex-specific incidence of 74.8 per 100,000. In 1937, the figure was 66.2 and in 1947, 72.6. The increase is under a modest 10%, and seems to confirm the conclusion that breast cancer morbidity and mortality in the United States have remained fairly constant during the past 3 decades.

There are no important relationships of breast cancer to socioeconomic levels. The more privileged classes have slightly more breast cancer than poorer women. These data also indicate that exogenous environmental factors are not major determinants in breast cancer. WYNDER [31] presents a relationship of breast cancer to dietary intake of oils and fats, a postulation deserving further study. Ionizing radiation [15] may increase breast cancer risk; there is association with the use of tobacco.

There is a minor (1.1 to 1) but consistently higher frequency of cancer of the left breast than of the right breast. This intriguing observation has no explanation, other than that the two breasts obviously are not identical, and probably has little practical significance. Of more importance is that cancer of the breast is often bilateral. The

life-time risk of cancer in the remaining breast in a woman who has lost one to cancer
is increased sixfold over the risk of the general population. In the United States, this
life-time risk is approximately 5%, or 1 of each 19 women; for those with cancer of
one breast, the risk for the other breast is 30%. Risk is a dynamic process, and
changes with age, as shown by ROBBINS and BERG [22].

Etiologic postulations concerning breast cancer can be divided into 4 major components: (a) reproductive physiology, (b) endogenous and exogenous hormones, (c)
viruses, and (d) genetic factors.

Relation to Reproduction

BERNARDINO RAMAZZINI, of Padua, the father of occupational medicine, in 1700
recorded that breast cancer was particularly common among nuns. He attributed the
situation to their celibate life style. To the obvious association of breast cancer to the
feminine gender was added association with the single state and nulliparity.

During the nineteenth century anecdotal descriptions in medicine began to be
replaced with quantitation. DOMENICO RIGONI-STERN in 1844 tabulated and analyzed
cancer mortality data from Verona. He showed clearly the increasing rate of breast
cancer with age, and the greater rate among single women, especially nuns. He won-
dered whether diet, compression of the breast by clothes or by praying positions
could be of importance, and he urged investigation of all religious orders, especially
since his four male breast cancers were among priests [24].

A long list of papers during the past century attests to the influences of reproductive physiology upon the occurrence of breast cancer. Although these influences
are real and reproducible, none of them exceeds a twofold effect upon risk as
compared with appropriate controls [27, 31].

Table 2. Relative risks to breast cancer. From SHAPIRO et al. [27]

Characteristic	Relative risk
Never married, vs. married	2.3
Pregnancies, 1—2 vs. 3 or more	2.0
Menarche, under 12 yrs. vs. over 15 yrs.	1.7
Menstruation, 30 yrs. or more vs. less than 30 yrs.	1.4
Breast conditions, 1 or more vs. none	3.1
Sisters, 1 or more with breast cancer vs. none	1.9

The outstanding prospective study by SHAPIRO et al. [27], of the Health Insurance
Plan of New York on the value of X-ray mammography in the detection of breast
cancer at more curable stages of the disease, also provides comparative risks of
various subpopulations identified by menarche, pregnancy, menopause and other
reproductive features. Table 2 summarizes these data.

Cancer of the breast, therefore, favors the single, nulliparous woman with an
early onset of menstruation and late menopause. It still remains to establish the

calculus of combining these factors, although interesting empirical approaches have been suggested [3].

A convincing number of well-designed studies demonstrate that lactation is not an important determinant in breast cancer [14, 17, 31]. Transgression against the ancient ethic for breast feeding of infants is not punished by mammary cancer, whatever else it may or may not lead to.

Preceding disease of the breast, such as the vague states grouped under "chronic cystic mastitis," is related to a threefold increase in risk to breast cancer [12, 27]. This finding should not be extrapolated to calling such abnormalities "precancerous." Intraductal papilloma, however, appears to fulfill the criteria for such designation. Analysis of data on X-ray mammograms and serial breast biopsies should lead to better understanding of the sequences of neoplastic development in the female breast. The novel microcatheterization of the breast, developed by OTTO SARTORIUS of Santa Barbara, has intriguing possibilities. As in many other neoplasms, the process of breast cancer is often multicentric and bilateral, and arises (or, really, becomes manifested) in tissues that are undergoing involution.

In the model case-control inquiry published in 1926 by JANET LANE-CLAYPON [12], there was a definite association of breast cancer to recalled history of trauma. The frequency of more objective evidence of trauma, such as laceration or suppuration, was not significantly different, leading to the conclusion of better or exaggerated recall among women whose attention was naturally more focused on their breast than that of the controls.

Relation to Hormones

The ameliorative effect of oophorectomy in premenopausal women with advanced cancer of the breast was reported by GEORGE BEATSON of London in 1896. It is one of the classics of cancer research.

The relationship of breast cancer to reproduction and to ovarian hormones also became clear from investigations on mice, as those published in 1919 by LEO LOEB of St. Louis.

HERRELL [9] in 1937 reported that the history of oophorectomy was elicited 10 times more frequently in women without cancer of the breast than in women with cancer of the breast (15 vs. 1.5%). Subsequent studies have borne out the protective role of oophorectomy, or, indeed, of early "natural" menopause.

The obverse, of increased cancer following prolonged exogenous exposure to estrogens, has been harder to prove. The data on women are moot, and retrospective studies on males with breast cancer also fail to reveal a relationship [23]. As an exception, perhaps, breast cancer has been reported in several transsex males remade into pseudo-females by surgical and chemical measures [30].

The carcinogenic effects of estrogens, so easily demonstrable in mice and in rats, has a more subtle expression in man. Women who were given an orally effective estrogen, diethylstilbestrol, to salvage their pregnancy have daughters who develop vaginal carcinoma [8]. The pregnancy-salvage therapy is now considered worthless. This thalidomide-like neoplastic effect on the fetus has yet to be expressed in the male progeny.

Many attempts have been made, in man and in the mouse, to relate breast cancer to a deviant hormonal state, usually an excess production of estrogenic components of the steroid hormones. The data are not convincing, and the concept is probably simplistic. In any case, the "determinants" of BULBROOK and his group [4] in England are still in the lead and point to subnormal levels of the androgenic components of the steroid constellation rather than increased estrogens. Their prospective studies, so appropriately being conducted on the Isle of Guernsey, bear continued watching. (Perhaps not so appropriately, since I have never heard of breast cancer in a cow.) Increasing attention is being directed at protein hormones, especially prolactin.

Levels of steroid byproducts in the urine, or even steroid levels of the conjugates in the blood, are rather peripheral to the site of neoplastic action, the reacting cell. The beautiful work of ELWOOD JENSEN [11] of Chicago on estrogen receptors in mammary gland cells, and the relation of such receptors to clinical response to hormones, is much closer to the target, and should be a prototype of a wider approach. Epidemiology of the future must include tissue studies as well as blood serum determinations.

Relation to Viruses

Only a few years ago, viruses as causes of cancer simply were not allowed in many orthodox cancer laboratories. Now they are front-stage center. Only a few years ago, the monumental discovery of the milk-transmitted virus in mice that caused breast cancer was considered a laboratory curiosity of mouse doctors playing with abnormal homozygous animals. Now the bandwagon is in the other direction. Claims and announcements are coming so rapidly that they are being made through newspapers rather than through scientific journals.

In any case, the target is the entity known as the "milk factor" of mice to some of us, as the Bittner virus to virologists favoring eponyms, as Type B Particle to electron microscopists, and now as the RNA-dependent DNA polymerase, nicknamed "reverse transcriptase" to biochemists.

It is an exciting era indeed, and I share in the enthusiasm but urge caution. Experience has shown already that oncogenic RNA viruses are hard to grow and harvest in any quantity, and that the transmission in man and in the rat is not as conveniently simple as it is in the mouse. In fact, I know of no convincing evidence that the RNA virus is involved in the rat mammary carcinoma. In the rat, breast cancers are induced by exposing them to polycyclic-hydrocarbon carcinogens, as the late HARRY SHAY [28] of Philadelphia, and CHARLES HUGGINS [10] of Chicago discovered. This is another story, of course, but it is appropriate to reiterate that the mouse and the rat continue to be informative experimental materials well worth research investment.

Relation to Heredity

It is well documented that breast cancer shows some familial aggregation. As with its other determinants, the aggregation is a mild one [14, 31]. Yet it can be said with some assurance that a woman is up to double the risk to breast cancer, as compared to the general population, if her history includes breast cancer in the mother, aunts or sisters.

Such aggregation, of course, does not have to be on a genetic basis. It may represent, in part or in whole, a comity of dietary and other habits, or shared environment.

Genetic aspects of breast cancer recently have had an important impetus from the investigations of NICHOLAS PETRAKIS [20, 21] of San Francisco. There is a relationship of breast cancer to the type of cerumen, a genetic trait. The relationship of ear wax to breast cancer is not as quixotic as it first appears. Cerumen and milk are specialized secretions produced by modified apocrine glands. The other relationship elicited by PETRAKIS is the admixture of white genetic material into black genetic pool, as measured by the Duffy gene. The data intimate that among the gifts of the whites to the blacks by such admixture is an increased susceptibility to breast cancer.

The important point of these investigations, as in the work on estrogen receptors, is that even epidemiology has entered the era of molecular biology. Conversely, epidemiology has contributions to make to molecular biology. And the gold of discovery lies at the interface!

Other Statistical Considerations

We can spin out the numbers game into various subrubrics of the breast cancer problem. Such studies do yield additional information, some of which may even be important.

There is a series of papers on the epidemiology of survival in breast cancer, such as the contributions of CUTLER et al. [5], relating various clinical and pathologic characteristics to life expectancy. The epidemiology of various histologic types of breast cancer has been touched upon by MAUSNER et al. [16] and by BERG and ROBBINS [22]. The epidemiology of metastases in breast cancer is still an unexplored field, although autopsy collections do exist [13] and could be related to clinical and demographic features. Such analyses require analytical sophistication and are full of traps for the unwary, such as selection of appropriate controls.

In the general area of numerical data on breast cancer, I commend to you 3 reports that are recent and reliable: LILIENFELD [14], DE WAARD [6] and the compilation by SEIDMAN [26]. The proceedings of the two national conferences on breast cancer, published in the December 1969 and December 1971 issues of *Cancer*, are chock-full of epidemiologic and other goodies.

L'Envoy

The quickening pace of cancer research promises interesting developments in the future. Yet one wonders whether some of our present hypotheses are but new terms for humours, miasma, ferments and constitution of three centuries ago.

Postulations must be built around the framework of objective facts. Astute observers who clearly distinguish facts from projections are rare at any age. One such man was CLAUDE GENDRON who in 1700 published his "Recherches sur la nature et la guerison des cancers" [19].

To GENDRON, cancer was a localized, resectable entity, spreading later with filaments and becoming adherent and incurable. He admitted ignorance as to causes but insisted that simple mechanical considerations of invasion, pressure and ulceration explained many of the manifestations without involving acid ferments.

Gendron's words on one patient with breast cancer (the mother of Louis XIV, the Sun King of France) retain currency and, alas, only too much relevance:

"When the Queen Mother Ann of Austria developed a lump in her left breast, my Uncle, the late Abbott Gendron, was summoned to the Royal Palace. He examined her, and he informed the King that the lump was an adherent, incurable cancer moreover on the verge of ulcerating ...

"But as members of the Royal Household could not tolerate the idea that incurable diseases should ever befall crowned heads, through intrigue and otherwise they managed to attract to the Palace workers of miracles. The latter promised the cure

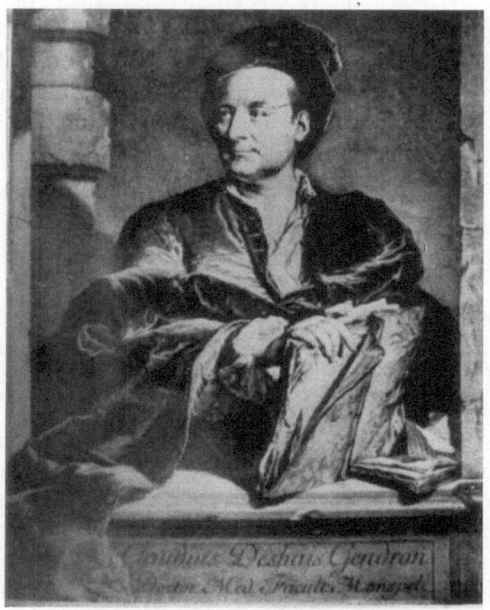

Fig. 2. Claude Deshais Gendron (1663—1750)
From Mustacchi and Shimkin [19]

of the cancer with so much confidence that many thought it strange that the health of the Queen should be entrusted to someone who had declared her incurable and did nothing but endeavor to prolong her life, while there were others who promised a perfect cure.

"... The King discharged my Uncle ... and ... my Uncle gave to the King a written account on what would be the effects of this so-called secret drug, a remedy well-known to him for a number of years. And, without fail, the Queen did develop every single complication my Uncle had predicted, so that everyone could see, though too late, there was a difference between him who bookishly drew his methods of treatment from the works of Paracelsus and ... my Uncle who because of his long experience had relied mostly on his own better understanding of the disease ...

"The cure of a disease, labeled incurable by those who master the Art of Healing, is not the privilege of those who excel in the practice of deception."

References

1. BERG, J. W., ROBBINS, G. F.: The histologic epidemiology of breast cancer. pp. 19—26. In Breast Cancer: Early and Late. M. D. Anderson 13th annual clinical conference on cancer, 1968. Chicago: Year Book Med. Publ. 1970.

2. Biometry Branch, National Cancer Institute, Preliminary Report Third National Cancer Survey 1969 Incidence. 1971.

3. BIRSNER, J. W., GERSHEN, C. J.: A diagnostic scoring system for breast cancer. Acta radiol. (in press).

4. BULBROOK, R. D., HAYWARD, J. L., ALLEN, D. S.: Further observations on steroid excretion and subsequent breast cancer in Guernsey. In: J. H. DE BUSSY (Ed.), Hormonal aspects in the epidemiology of human breast cancer. pp. 163—170. Amsterdam 1969.

5. CUTLER, S. J., CHRISTINE, B., BARCLAY, T. H. C.: Increasing incidence and decreasing mortality rates for breast cancer. Cancer (Philad.) 28, 1376—1380 (1971).

6. DE WAARD, F.: The epidemiology of breast cancer; review and prospects. Int. J. Cancer 4, 577—586 (1969).

7. DOLL, R., MUIR, C. WATERHOUSE, J. (Eds.): Cancer Incidence in Five Continents. pp. 388, Vol. II. New York: Springer 1970.

8. HERBST, A. L., ULFELDER, H., POSKANZER, D. C.: Adenocarcinoma of the vagina: association of maternal stilbestrol therapy with tumor appearance in young women. New. Engl. J. Med. 284, 878—881 (1971).

9. HERRELL, W. E.: The relative incidence of oophorectomy in women with and without carcinoma of the breast. Amer. J. Cancer 29, 659—665 (1937).

10. HUGGINS, C., BRISIARELLI, G., SUTTON, H., JR.: Rapid induction of mammary carcinoma in the rat and the influence of hormones on the tumors. J. exp. Med. 109, 25—42 (1959).

11. JENSEN, E. V., NUMATA, M., BRECHER, P. I., DESOMBRE, E. R.: Hormone-receptor interaction as a guide to biochemical mechanism. Biochem. Soc. Symp. 32, 133—159 (1971).

12. LANE-CLAYPON, J. E.: A further report on cancer of the breast, with special references to its associated antecedent conditions. Repts. Min. Health No. 32. London 1926.

13. LEVSHIN, V. F.: Metastases of cancer of the mammary gland on data from autopsies. Vop. Onkol. 16, 7, 23—28 (1970).

14. LILIENFELD, A.: The epidemiology of breast cancer. Cancer Res. 23, 1503—1513 (1963).

15. MacKENZIE, I.: Breast cancer following multiple fluoroscopies. Brit. J. Cancer 9, 1—18 (1965).

16. MAUSNER, J. S., SHIMKIN, M. B., MOSS, N. H., ROSEMOND, G. P.: Cancer of the breast in Philadelphia hospitals 1951—1964. Cancer (Philad.) 23, 260—274 (1969).

17. MIRRA, A. P., COLE, P., MacMAHON, B.: Breast cancer in an area of high parity; Sao Paulo, Brazil. Cancer Res. 31, 77—83 (1971).

18. MOULTON, F. R. (Ed.): A Symposium on Mammary Tumors in Mice. Washington: Amer. Ass. Ad. Sci. 1945.

19. MUSTACCHI, P., SHIMKIN, M. B.: Gendron's enquiries into the nature, knowledge and cure of cancers. Cancer (Philad.) 9¹ 644—647 (1965).

20. PETRAKIS, N. L.: Cerumen genetics and human breast cancer. Science 173, 347—349 (1971).

21. PETRAKIS, N. L.: Some preliminary observations on the influence of genetic admixture on cancer incidence in American Negroes. Inst. J. Cancer 7, 256—258, 8, 184 (1971).

22. ROBBINS, G. F., BERG, J. W.: Bilateral primary breast cancers. Cancer (Philad.) 17, 1501—1527 (1964).

23. SCHOTTENFIELD, D., LILIENFELD, A. M., DIAMOND, H.: Some observations on the epidemiology of breast cancer among males. Amer. J. publ. Hlth 53, 890—897 (1963).

24. SCOTTO, J., BAILAR, J. C. III: Rigoni-Stern and medical statistics. J. Hist. Med. allied Sci. 24, 65—75 (1969).

25. SEGI, M.: Cancer Mortality for Selected Sites in 24 Countries (1950—1957). Dept. Publ. Health, Tohoku U. Sch. Med. Sendai, Japan 1960.

26. SEIDMAN, H.: Cancer of the breast. Statistical and epidemiological data. New York: Amer. Cancer Soc. Inc. 1969.

27. Shapiro, S., Strax, P., Venet, L., Fink, R.: The search for risk factors in breast cancer. Amer. J. publ. Hlth **58**, 820—835 (1968).
28. Shay, H., Aegerter, E. A., Gruenstein, M., Komarov, S. A.: Development of adenocarcinoma of the breast in the Wistar rat following the gastric instillation of methylcholanthrene. J. nat. Cancer Inst. **10**, 255—266 (1949).
29. Shimkin, M. B.: Cancer of the breast. Some old facts and new perspectives. J. Amer. med. Ass. **183**, 358—361 (1963).
30. Symmers, W. S.: Carcinoma of the breast in transsexual individuals after surgical and hormonal interference with the primary and secondary sex characteristics. Brit. med. J. **11**, 82—85 (1968).
31. Wynder, E. L.: Identification of women at high risk for breast cancer. Cancer (Philad.) **24**, 1235—1240 (1969).
An excellent review is by Brian MacMahon et al. J. Nat. Cancer Inst. **50**, 21—42 (1973).

Viral Transmission in Breast Cancer*

N. H. Sarkar and D. H. Moore

Breast cancer is widely distributed among different species of mammals, including humans. At one time the disease was considered to be hereditary, especially in women, because of familial clustering [1]. As early as 1907, Borrel [2] speculated upon the possibility of a viral etiology for cancer in general, but to date no definite evidence of viral involvement in breast cancer has been found other than in mice. The definitive proof of the viral etiology of a disease is obtained when it satisfies Koch's postulates, i.e. the suspected virus is encountered in every case of the disease and preparations of the virus on injections to proper hosts cause the disease. The virus involved in mouse mammary tumors has satisfied Koch's postulates and thus has been accepted as the causative agent. Breast cancer in mice has been studied in an attempt to develop a rational approach to the study of breast cancer in other species, particularly human.

Some evidence has now accumulated suggesting viral involvement in monkey and rat mammary tumors, and possibly in human mammary tumors. We shall first review the viral etiology of breast cancer in mice and then the situation in monkeys, rats, and humans.

Mouse Mammary Tumor Virus (MuMTV)

In 1911 Murray [3] observed that female mice whose mothers or grandmothers had cancer of the breast were distinctly more susceptible to spontaneous development of the disease than those in whose ancestry cancer incidence was more remote. In mating experiments, Murray and Little [4, 5] found a considerably higher incidence of tumors among the offspring of high tumor females and low tumor males than among the offspring of low tumor females and high tumor males, indicating that mammary cancer in mice is influenced by extrachromosomal, as well as genetic factors.

Using inbred strains of mice Bittner [6] discovered that the 88% incidence of mammary tumors in strain A mice dropped to 33% when these mice were foster nursed by low tumor CBA strain mothers. Additional evidence for an extrachromosomal "milk factor" was thus indicated. Subsequently Bittner [7], and others [8—10] found tumorigenic activity in extracts of tumors from high cancer strain mice. Thus it

* Supported by Contract PH 43-68-1000 within the Special Virus Cancer Program of the N.C.I., National Institutes of Health, U.S. Public Health Service Grant CA-08740 from N.C.I., General Research Support Grant FR-5582 from N.C.I. and Grant-in-Aid M-43 from the State of New Jersey.

became evident that both milk and tumors contained some agent that could produce breast cancer in mice.

The work of Porter and Thomson [11], Graff et al. [12], and Passey et al. [13] indicated a correlation between the presence of particles of varying sizes as revealed by electron microscopy in tumor extracts and the latter's ability to induce tumors.

During the 1950's Bernhard [14] and others [15—19] demonstrated two types of particles in thin sections of mammary tumors. Bernhard described the intracytoplasmic particles (65—75 mμ in diameter) as type A and the extracellular particles (100—120 mμ in diameter) as type B [14]. To prove that these B particles were responsible for the induction of mammary tumors many investigators attempted to isolate and determine the tumorigenicity of these particles. Improved methods of purification [20], identification by electron microscopy, and more rapid assay procedures were developed [21]. Finally, by titrations of infective fractions, a correlation was found between infectivity and a specific particle, the B particle [21—24]. The main route of transmission of the disease from mother to offspring is through milk. However, the experimental results of Andervont and Dunn [25], Foulds [26], Mühlbock [27], Bittner and Frantz [28], Bittner [29] and Andervont [30], have made it clear that some high-breast-cancer strains male mice can also infect agent-free females with which they mate.

Mammary tumor virus activity has also been detected in the blood of various MuMTV-carrying strains of mice (for details see references [31, 32]). Both the blood cells and the plasma were shown to contain B particles and bioactivity. Thus the correlation between the presence of B particles and the ability to induce mammary tumors in mice is very extensive.

Adenomas, later called hyperplastic alveolar nodules, were recognized and described in the beginning of this century (see reference [33]). They were considered to be pre-neoplastic structures. Mammary tumors arise more frequently and earlier from transplanted nodule outgrowths than from normal tissue outgrowths. Thus it seems logical that B particles transform normal cells into nodule cells which in turn are transformed into neoplastic cells. The virus may be involved in both transformations. After removing the milk-transmitted virus from C3H mice by foster nursing, B particles are still found in the tumors which develop late in the life of these animals. These mice also develop many nodules which contain B particles. However, injection of cell-free extracts of either the nodules or the late-developing tumors shows no bioactivity. This agent which is transmitted by male or female parents to their progeny, even in the absence of nursing, has been called nodule-inducing virus (NIV). This is a misnomer because the milk transmitted virus is a better producer of nodules than is NIV. Investigators differ in their views regarding the presence or absence of B particles in the tumors and milk of low-cancer strains where the tumors appear very late in life. When B particles have been demonstrated in such strains their significance has been questioned.

There are many complex aspects of mammary tumorigenesis in the mouse, including dependency on genetics, hormonal involvement, immune response and strain susceptibility. The wide variation in the spontaneous mammary tumor incidence and the age at which the tumors appear in mice are illustrated in Table 1. The variation in susceptibility of several strains and F_1-hybrids to inoculations of the same virus is shown in Table 2. The widespread distribution of leukemia virus(es) in different

Table 1. Incidence of spontaneous mammary tumor and leukemia in different strains of mice in our colony

Strain	Percentage of animals with mammary tumors at different ages			Percentage of Leukemia [a]
	12 months	24 months	Average age of tumor development in months	
A	98	99	11	0
Af	2.7	50	18.5	21
BALB/c	3.5	28	20.2	22
BALB/cf C3H	97	97	7.1	2
C57BL/Haag/f C57BL/He	0	0	—	17
C57BL/Haag	0	0	—	24
DBA-RIII	98	98	7.3	0
GR	99	99	7.1	6
RIII	96	96	9	0
RIIIf/He	0	5	16	4

[a] Recorded at autopsy from observation of enlarged spleen, liver, thymus and/or lymph nodes.

Table 2. Susceptibility of some inbred mouse strains and their F_1-hybrids to purified mammary tumor virus from C3H mouse milk

Recipient strain or hybrid	Mice with tumors [a] / mice at risk (%) Dilutions of a stock virus				
	10^{-2}	10^{-3}	10^{-4}	10^{-5}	10^{-6}
BALB/c	9/10 (90)	25/30 (83)	41/50 (82)	15/27 (56)	10/22 (45)
C3Hf	16/20 (80)	8/16 (50)	11/21 (52)	3/13 (23)	0/31 (0)
(C3HfxBALB/c)F₁	12/14 (86)	16/25 (64)	14/15 (93)	8/13 (62)	2/10 (20)
(020xBALB/c)F₁	12/20 (60)	35/45 (78)	13/25 (52)	4/38 (11)	0/43 (0)
(C57BLxC3Hf)F₁	5/10 (50)	18/32 (56)	13/37 (35)	2/11 (18)	0/19 (0)
(C3Hfx020)F₁	15/31 (48)	13/24 (54)	1/25 (4)	0/36 (0)	0/22 (0)
(C57BLxBALB/c)F₁	9/13 (69)	12/20 (60)	2/19 (11)	1/36 (3)	0/15 (0)

[a] Mammary Tumor Incidence at One Year [24].

Table 3. Potency of the mammary tumor virus to tumor development and the modes of vertical transmission

Virus	Mouse strain	Modes of vertical transmission [a]		
		Milk	Ovum	Sperm
Virulent	C3H	+++	—	+
Plaque forming virus	GR	+++	+++	+++
Low oncogenic	C3Hf	+	++	++
Very low oncogenic	BALB/c	—	++	++

[a] — indicates no transmission, + incidental transmission, ++ always transmission but not always manifestation, +++ always transmission and manifestation.

strains (Table 1) has further complicated mammary tumor virus research. It is now recognized [24] that there are at least 4 different morphologically indistinguishable strains of the virus, which differ (with overlaps) in virulence and mode of transmission (Table 3).

Although the viral etiology of mammary tumors in mice has been established through biological experimentation, clearly such tests are out of the question for any suspected agent in human breast tumors. Thus the morphological, biochemical and immunological aspects of any suspected agent in humans must be explored in detail using the mouse virus as a model. The following are characteristic properties of the mouse mammary tumor virus.

A. Morphological

Mature mouse mammary tumor virus (MuMTV) is a spherical, enveloped particle 100—120 mμ in diameter containing a spherical eccentric nucleoid which is also surrounded by a membrane. The viral membrane is covered with spikes, which are

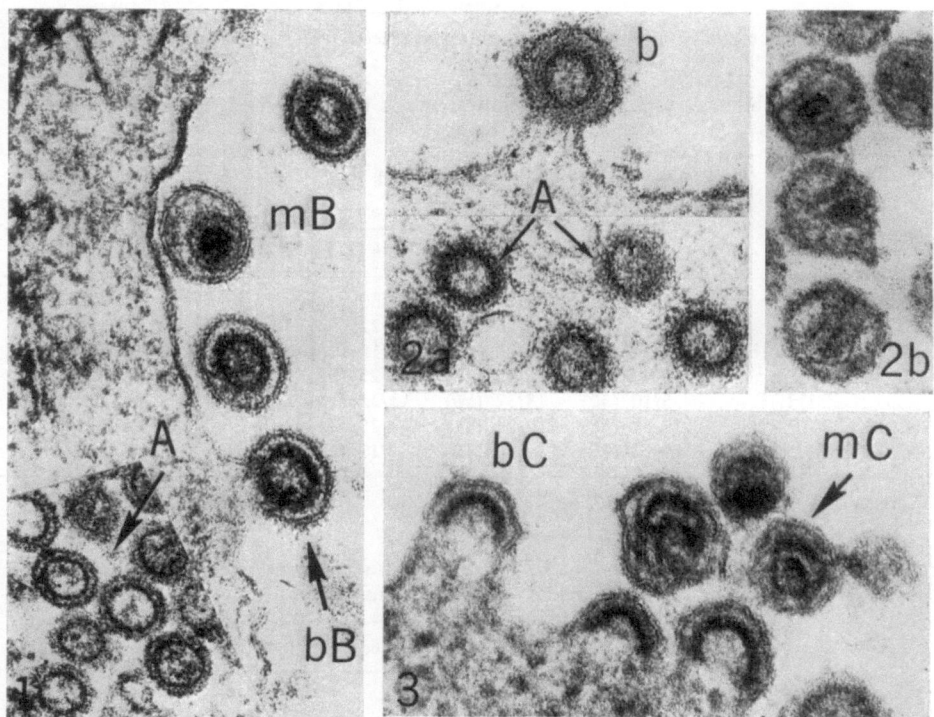

Fig. 1. Examples of intracytoplasmic A, budding B (bB) and mature mouse mammary tumor virus particles (mB). ×120,000

Fig. 2. Intracytoplasmic A and budding particles (b) in NC-37 cell infected with a virus (M-PMV) associated with a monkey mammary tumor (Fig. 2 a). The extracellular virus particles are shown in Fig. 2 b. ×120,000

Fig. 3. Budding (bC) and extracellular mature (mC) R-35 virus (Courtesy G. Schidlovsky of John L. Smith Memorial for Cancer Research, Pfizer, Inc.). ×120,000

often obscured in thin section preparations. Intracytoplasmic A particles are incorporated into the budding process to form mature particles (Fig. 1). The structure of the nucleoid is often found to be pleomorphic. In negative staining the virions usually show a head and tail configuration and the spikes are well resolved (Fig. 4). They are 98 Å long, consisting of a thin stalk with 50 Å knob at the distal end. Individual spikes are spaced 73 Å center to center and are surrounded by either five

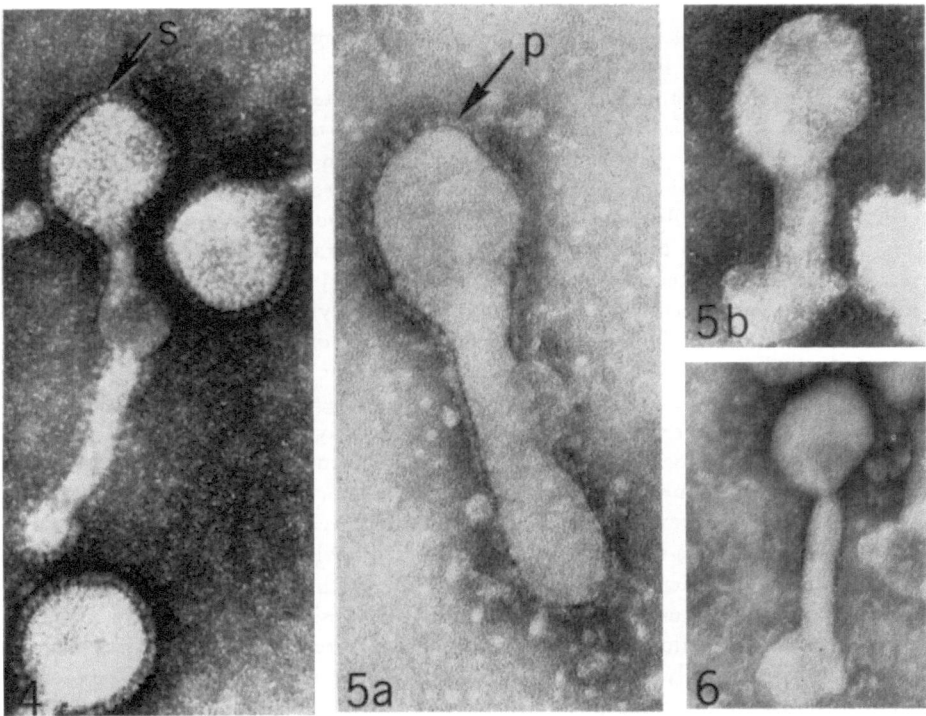

Figs. 4—6. Negatively stained micrographs of MuMTV (Fig. 4), M-PMV (Fig. 5 a and 5 b) and R-35 virus (Fig. 6). Note the difference in structure of the spikes (S) of MuMTV and the projections (P) of M-PMV. The smooth viral membrane of M-PMV is shown in Fig. 5 b and R-35 in Fig. 6. Figs. 5 a and 6 from G. SCHIDLOVSKY. Fig. 4 and 5, ×170,000; Fig. 6, ×120,000

or six neighbors, the 6-fold symmetry predominating [34]. The structure of the characteristic spikes are different from the surface projections of the myxo, paramyxo and other viruses. They are also different from the projections of cellular membranes. Although the detailed structure of the nucleocapsid in most virions is obscured, single strands 30 Å in diameter and helical structures 70—90 Å in diameter can be observed [35]

B. Biochemical

The virions contain 60—70 S single stranded RNA, which is converted into 36—37 S components by heating or by treatment with dimethylsulfoxide [36].

Reverse transcriptase (RTase): An enzyme, RNA dependent DNA polymerase, that mediates the synthesis of DNA, using single-stranded viral RNA as a template, has been found in MuMTV [37]. The existence of this enzyme, discovered by Temin and Mizutani [38] and Baltimore [39] is a unique characteristic of all the oncogenic RNA viruses. The DNA product is complementary to viral RNA and hybridizes specifically with it.

C. Viral Proteins and Antigens

Polyacrylamide gel electrophoresis of MuMTV shows five major polypeptides in the virions [40]. The molecular weights of these are: p1 (90,000), p2 (70,000), p3 (52,000), p4 (33,000) and p5 (23,000). The major protein of the virus is p3 which is a constituent of the viral nucleoid. Protein p5 is the structural protein of the membrane. Tween 80-ether treatment of MuMTV results in disruption of the viral membrane and release of the viral nucleoid [34]. Prolonged lipid extraction with detergents results in virtually complete solubilization of the virions and the soluble proteins can be separated by Sephadex G-200 chromatography. Antibodies produced in rats against these proteins identify five viral antigens [40]. Two antigens have been found to be group-specific and are the antigens of the viral nucleoid. They are found in virus derived from the milk and mammary tumors of C3H, DBA/2, A, RIII, GR and Swiss Ha/ICR mice. These antigens are also present in nodules of DBA/2f, C3Hf, Af and (Balb ♀×C3H ♂)F$_1$ mice. Thus there are antigenic similarities of the viruses obtained from different strains of mice, and only recently strain-specificity of MuMTV antigens has been observed [41]. It has been demonstrated that sera from mice immunized against MuMTV can neutralize the biological activity of the virus [42]. More recently Charney and Moore [43] have succeeded in completely protecting C57BL (MuMTV-free) mice against a subsequent live virus challenge by a single dose of formaldehyde—inactivated, purified MuMTV. Both infection and tumorigenesis were prevented. Immunization of RIII (MuMTV-positive) mice did not result in abortion of the infection (these mice still secreted virus in their milk) but tumorigenesis was significantly delayed. Tween 80-ether disrupted virus can also be successfully used as an immunogen to protect C57BL mice against MuMTV infection (Sarkar and Moore, unpublished results).

It is interesting to note that the protein pattern of MuMTV differs from the proteins of the avian, murine, hamster and leukemia sarcoma viruses; furthermore, MuMTV is serologically unrelated to the leukemia-sarcoma viruses [44].

Suspected Breast Cancer Viruses

As has been mentioned earlier, the most direct proof that breast cancer is of viral origin is to demonstrate the ability of the cell-free filtrates of tumors to transmit the disease from one animal to another of the same or related species. Besides direct transmission, the studies of MuMTV and leukemia-sarcoma viruses (C particles) suggest that these viruses have several characteristic properties in common [45] which can serve as diagnostic indications for any suspected oncogenic RNA tumor virus. These are: 1. Characteristic structure as revealed by electron microscopy. Budding and extracellular particles morphologically similar to B or C particles found in tumor cells would be indicative of oncornavirions. The characteristic difference in surface morphology of B and C particles as revealed by negative staining could further define the type of particle. Furthermore, helical nucleocapsid structure of the particle would place it into the oncorna group. 2. Detection of 60—70 S RNA and 3. RNA-dependent DNA polymerase would confirm the viral nature of the suscepted particles to be oncorna type. 4. Another means of testing a suspected tumor virus would be to determine the relationship of its nucleic acid to that of other known tumor viruses by measuring the degree of hybridization between the known and the suspected virus. 5. Similarity of the protein pattern of isolated particles to those of leukemia-sarcoma viruses and murine mammary tumor viruses may prove to be of considerable use in identifying prospective oncornaviruses. 6. Antigenic similarity of the unknown viruses to known viruses could also be helpful. It should be mentioned however, that the criterions 4—6 may or may not be exactly fulfilled with the suspected viruses. They may have different protein composition and they may be biochemically and anti-genically unrelated to known viruses.

1. Monkey Mammary Tumor Virus (M-PMV)

A mammary carcinoma that arose spontaneously in an eight year old rhesus monkey at the Mason Research Institute was found by electron microscopy to contain a large number of particles resembling oncorna viruses [46]. The presence of intra-cytoplasmic A particles in virus-producing cells and its incorporation into budding particles (Fig. 2) is morphologically similar to the characteristic budding phenomenon of B particles, In negative staining the membranes of most particles appear smooth (Fig. 5 b) like leukemia-sarcoma viruses; this is in contrast to the (98 Å long) spike-covered surface of murine mammary tumor virus. However, a small number of particles ($< 5^0/0$) show short (50 Å long) projections on the viral membrane (Fig. 5 a). The structure of the nucleoid is more pleomorphic (Fig. 2 b) than those of the B and C particles. Thus, although these particles do not clearly fit into the category of B or C type morphology, they do have certain similarities. However, the antisera pre-pared against Tween 80-ether disrupted M-PMV do not react with the known oncornaviruses; neither do ether-treated virions react in immuno-diffusion tests with potent antisera prepared against the group-specific antigens of the known oncorna-viruses [47]. A clear serologic relationship between M-PMV and known oncorna viruses has thus not been demonstrated.

The close evolutionary relationship between man and monkey and the ability of M-PMV to grow in rhesus monkey embryo cells, human lymphocytes and in monkey and chimpanzee lung cell lines stimulated interest in the possible relationship of M-PMV to the causative agent of human carcinomas. Unfortunately, immunodiffusion tests using anti-M-PMV sera failed to detect M-PMV antigens in human carcinomas of breast, rectum, squamous cell, kidney, embryo, ovary, colon and stomach or in human sarcomas, e. g. liposarcoma, osteogenic sarcoma, myxolipofibrosarcoma or leomyosarcoma as well as a wide variety of fetal and normal adult tissues [47].

This virus contains 60—70 S as well as 4 S RNA [47] and an RNA directed DNA polymerase [48]. Viral replication is inhibited by actinomycin D [47]. Although the tumorigenic potential of this virus is still unknown, certain properties of this virus fit those of the oncornaviruses, which increases the likelihood that this agent is an oncogenic RNA virus. Whether or not this virus will be shown to be a mammary cancer or leukemia virus remains to be seen.

2. Rat Mammary Tumor Virus (R-35)

A spontaneous mammary fibroadenoma of a Huggins rat gradually changed to mammary adenocarcinoma during prolonged serial transplantation in Sprague-Dawley female rats. Electron microscopic studies of the R-35 subline of this tumor revealed the presence of C-type virus particles [49]. An established cell line of this tumor in tissue culture was found to produce C-particles continuously. Cell-free preparations of R-35 virus can infect monolayer cell cultures (epithelial cells) originating from lactating rat mammary tissue [50]. Infected cells transform into discrete foci of hyperrefractile spindle and rounded cells, which show ultrastructural alteration of the nuclei, mitochondria, polyribosomes, endoplasmic reticulum and Golgi apparatus [50, 51]. These transformed cells only support the replication of C-type virus particles (Fig. 3). In the negatively stained preparations the particles show head and tail form; the viral membrane does not have surface projections (Fig. 6). The etiologic role of this virus in rat mammary tumors or leukemia and its antigenic relationship with other oncogenic viruses is still unknown.

3. Human Mammary Tumor Virus

A number of electron microscopic examinations of ultrathin sections of human breast tumor tissues have been made for the possible presence of virus-like particles (for details see references [52, 53, 54]). Some of these studies have reported the presence of particles which morphologically resemble mouse mammary tumor, or leukemia-sarcoma viruses. Examples of budding particles have also been observed. In thin section electron microscopy of human milk fractions, virus-like particles resembling B and or C type viruses have been found. However, due to the small number of isolated particles observed in these studies their identification is questionable, especially since similar structures of cellular origin are frequently observed. Recently we have found particles identical in morphology to B particles in negatively stained preparations of human milk isolates [52, 55—58]. These particles have been seen in 13 milk specimens out of 381 milk samples from American women (Table 4), and only 1 or 2 particles were found in each case after an extensive search. The particles show head and tail formation and have surface spikes similar in shape, size and distribution to those of the mouse B particles (Fig. 7). These particles have been designated as MS-1 type to differentiate them from mouse B particles [57, 58]. Furthermore, human milk also contains two other kinds of particles. One type (Figs. 8 and 9) has the overall size and shape of type MS-1 particles but the surface projections of these particles are not identical to those of type MS-1. These have been designated as type MS-2 particles. It is interesting to note that avian myeloblastosis and a few monkey mammary tumor virions (described earlier) also contain projections resembling MS-2 particles. The nature of MS-2 particles is unknown, but could possibly represent cellular fragments or type MS-1 in various stages of degradation or these are virus particles having different type of projections. MS-2 particles have been found in 41 specimens. Another type of particle (MS-3) is comprised of those similar in shape and size to MS-1 and MS-2 particles, having head and tail formation but no surface projections (Fig. 10). Thus MS-3 particles resemble negatively stained leukemia-sarcoma viruses, and the viruses that have been found to be associated with monkey and rat mammary tumor. These particles have appeared in 134 out of 381 specimens and in larger quantities than MS-1 and MS-2. Thin section electron micro-scopy of some of these samples revealed very few particles that resembled either B or C. Thus it is possible that most of the MS-3 particles seen by negative staining are cell debris; a few could be C type viruses.

It has been found very recently that a density gradient purified fraction of certain human milks exhibited reverse transcriptase activity [59]. Furthermore, some human milk fractions also contain 70 S RNA [60]. Such an enzyme activity and the presence

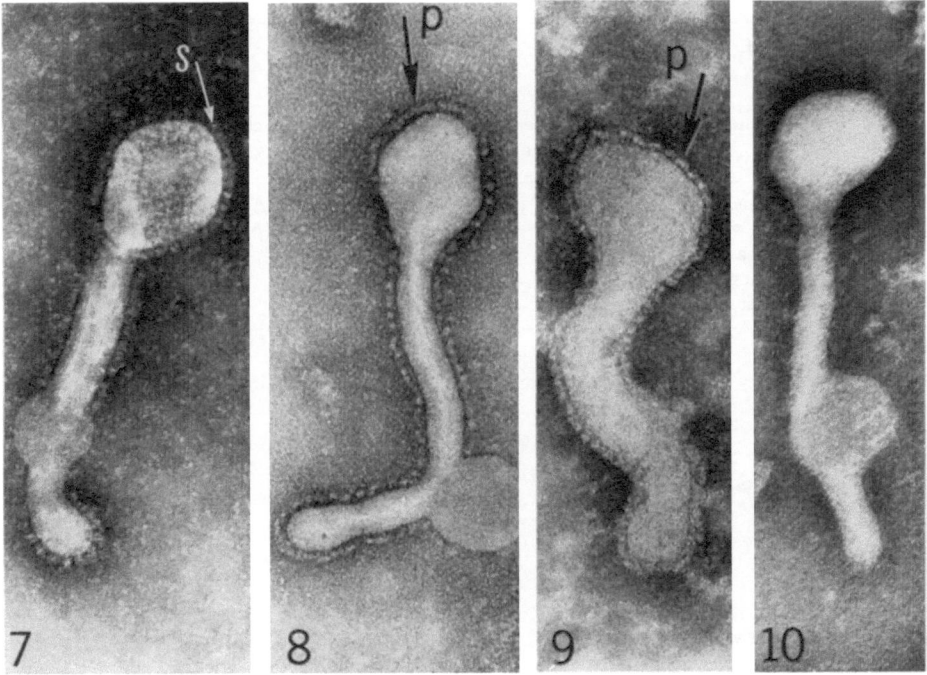

Figs. 7—10. Virus-like particles in human milk. The spikes (S) of the particle in Fig. 7 is identical to those of MuMTV (compare Fig. 7 with Fig. 4). The structure of the projections (P) of the particles in Figs. 8 and 9 are different than in Fig. 7. The particle in Fig. 10 has smooth membranes and resembles C-type viruses. ×175,000. Fig. 7 is from ref. [57]

of 70 S RNA are known to be a characteristic feature of the oncogenic RNA viruses. However, the presence of polymerase activity in those milks that contain one or more kinds of particles (Table 5), makes it difficult to determine which one of these par-ticles is associated with the reverse transcriptase. The morphological similarity of MS-1 particles in human milks to mouse B particles, the presence of neutralizing anti-body in some human sera that partially neutralizes the infectivity of mouse mammary tumor virus [61] and the homology of the MuMTV-RNA to the polysomal RNA extracted from human breast tumors [62] suggest the possibility that a MuMTV related virus may be present in human milk. One of the particles described above may thus be a candiate. A question arises as to the presence of these particles (Table 4) and polymerase activity (Table 5) in milks from women both with and without a

Table 4. Distribution of the three different types of virus-like particles in human milk [a]

Breast cancer history (maternal)	Number of women or specimens		Type of particles					
			MS-1		MS-2		MS-3	
History	# Women	90	4	4.4%	15	16.7%	33	36.7%
	# Specimen	133	4	3.0%	20	15.0%	45	33.8%
No history	# Women	173	9	5.2%	20	11.6%	69	39.9%
	# Specimen	248	9	3.6%	21	8.5%	89	35.9%

[a] Taken from ref. 57.

Table 5. Occurrence of the three different types of virus-like particles in human milk and the RNA-dependent DNA polymerase activity [a]

Milk samples from women with a family history of breast cancer	Type of particles			RNA-Dependent DNA-Polymerase
	MS-1	MS-2	MS-3	
1	−	+	+	+
2	−	−	+	+
3	−	−	+	+
4	−	−	−	−
5	−	+	+	−
6	−	−	+	−
7	−	−	−	−
8	−	−	−	−
9	+	+	+	+
10	−	−	−	−
Milk samples from women with no cancer nistory				
1	−	+	+	+
2	−	−	+	−
3	−	−	+	+
4	−	−	+	+
5	−	−	−	−
6	−	−	−	−
7	+	+	+	+
8	−	−	−	−
9	−	−	+	−
10	−	−	+	−

[a] Taken from ref. 57.

familial history (maternal) of breast cancer. The simplest assumption is that infection with the human mammary tumor agent is widespread and perhaps ubiquitous in women. Overt tumorigenesis in women carrying the infection would then depend upon additional genetic, hormonal and immunologic factors as indeed is the case in various mouse strains [24]. Infection may be due to exposure to the virus (e. g. by nursing or contact) or by vertical transmission through ovum or sperm; again as is the case in various strains of mice.

References

1. TOKUHATA, G. K.: Morbidity and mortality among offspring of breast cancer mothers. Amer. J. Epidem. 89, 139 (1969).
2. BORREL, A.: Le probleme du cancer revue. Bull. Inst. Pasteur 5, 497—512, 593—608, 641—662 (1907).
3. MURRAY, J. A.: Cancerous ancestry and the incidence of cancer in mice. Sci. Rep. Cancer Res. Fd (Lond.) 4, 114 (1911).
4. MURRAY, J. A.: The genetics of mammary tumor incidence in mice. Genetics 20, 466 (1935).
5. MURRAY, W. S., LITTLE, C. C.: Extrachromosomal influence of mammary and non-mammary tumors in mice. Amer. J. Cancer 27, 516 (1936).
6. BITTNER, J. J.: Some possible effects of nursing on mammary gland tumor incidence in mice. Science 84, 162 (1936).
7. BITTNER, J. J.: The preservation by freezing and drying in vacuo of the milk influence for the development of breast cancer in mice. Science 93, 527 (1941).
8. BRYAN, W. R., KAHLER, H., SHIMKIN, M. B., ANDERVONT, H. B.: Extraction and ultra-centrifugation of mammary tumor inciter in mice. J. nat. Cancer Inst. 2, 451 (1942).
9. VISSCHER, M. B., GREEN, R. G., BITTNER, J. J.: Characterization of the milk influence in spontaneous mammary carcinoma. Proc. Soc. exp. Biol. (N. Y.) 49, 94 (1942).
10. ANDERVONT, H. B., BRYAN, W. R.: Properties of the mouse mammary tumor agent. J. nat. Cancer Inst. 5, 143 (1944).
11. PORTER, K. R., THOMPSON, H. P.: A particulate body associated with epithelial cells cultured from mammary carcinomas of mice of a milk factor strain. J. exp. Med. 88, 15 (1948).
12. GRAFF, S., MOORE, D. H., STANLEY, W. M., RANDALL, H. T., HAAGENSEN, C. D.: Isolation of mouse mammary carcinoma virus. Cancer (Philad.) 2, 755 (1949).
13. PASSEY, R. D., DMOCHOWSKI, L., REED, R., ASTBURY, W. T.: Biophysical studies of extracts of tissues of high- and low-breast-cancer-strain mice. Biochim. et Biophys. Acta 4, 391 (1950).
14. BERNHARD, W.: Electron microscopy of tumor cells and tumor viruses: A review. Cancer Res. 18, 491 (1958).
15. DMOCHOWSKI, L., HAAGENSEN, C. D., MOORE, D. H.: Studies of sections of normal and malignant cells of high- and low-cancer strain mice by means of electron microscopy. Acta Un. int. Cancr. 11, 640 (1955).
16. BANG, F. B., ANDERVONT, H. B., VELLISTO, I.: Electron microscopic evidence concerning the mammary tumor inciter (virus). II. An electron microscopic study of spontaneous and induced mammary tumors of mice. Bull. Johns Hopk. Hosp. 98, 287 (1956 a).
17. BANG, F. B., VELLISTO, I., LIBERT, R.: Electron microscopic evidence concerning the mammary tumor inciter (virus). I. A study of normal and malignant cells from the mammary gland of mice. Bull. Johns Hopk. Hosp. 98, 255 (1956 b).
18. PITELKA, D. R., BERN, H. H., DE OME, K. B., SCHOOLEY, C. N., WELLINGS, S. R.: Virus-like particles in hyperplastic alveolar nodules of the mammary gland of the C3H/HeCRGL mouse. J. nat. Cancer Inst. 20, 541 (1958).
19. ICHIKAWA, Y., AMANO, S.: A new type of virus found in a spontaneous mammary tumor of SL mice and its proliferating modus observed in ultra-thin sections under the electron microscope. Gann 49, 57 (1958).
20. LYONS, M. J., MOORE, D. H.: Isolation of the mouse mammary tumor virus: chemical and morphological studies. J. nat. Cancer Inst. 35, 549 (1965).
21. CHARNEY, J., PULLINGER, B. D., MOORE, D. H.: Development of an infectivity assay for mouse mammary tumor virus. J. nat. Cancer Inst. 43, 1289 (1969).

22. Hageman, P. C., Links, J., Bentvelzen, P.: Biological properties of B particles from C3H and C3Hf mouse milk. J. nat. Cancer Inst. **40**, 1319 (1968).
23. Moore, D. H., Pillsbury, N., Pullinger, B. D.: Titrations of mammary tumor virus in fresh and treated RIII milk and milk fractions. J. nat. Cancer Inst. **43**, 1263 (1969).
24. Bentvelzen, P., Daams, J. H., Hageman, P., Calafat, J.: Genetic transmission of viruses that incite mammary tumor in mice. Proc. nat. Acad. Sci. (Wash.) **67**, 377 (1970).
25. Andervont, H. B., Dunn, T. B.: Mammary tumors in mice presumably free of the mammary tumor agent. J. nat. Cancer Inst. **8**, 227 (1948).
26. Foulds, L.: Mammary tumor in hybrid mice: the presence and transmission of the mammary tumor agent. Brit. J. Cancer **3**, 230 (1949).
27. Mühlbock, O.: Studies on the transmission of the mouse mammary tumor agent by the male parent. J. nat. Cancer Inst. **12**, 819 (1952).
28. Bittner, J. J., Frantz, M. J.: Sensitivity of females of the C stock to male infection with the mammary tumor agent. Proc. Soc. exp. Biol. (N. Y.) **86**, 698 (1954).
29. Bittner, J. J.: Influence of the mammary-tumor agent on the genesis of mammary cancer in agent-free mouse after male transmission. J. nat. Cancer Inst. **25**, 177 (1960).
30. Andervont, H. B.: *In utero* transmission of the mouse mammary tumor agent. J. nat. Cancer Inst. **31**, 261 (1963).
31. Nandi, S.: The histocompatibility-2 locus and susceptibility to Bittner virus borne by red blood cells in mice. Proc. nat. Acad. Sci. (Wash.) **58**, 485 (1967).
32. Moore, D. H., Sarkar, N. H., Charney, J.: Bioactivity and virions in the blood of mice with mammary tumor virus. J. nat. Cancer Inst. **44**, 965 (1970).
33. Nandi, S., de Ome, K. B.: An interference phenomenon associated with resistance to infection with mouse mammary tumor virus. J. nat. Cancer Inst. **35**, 299 (1965).
34. Sarkar, N. H., Nowinski, R. C., Moore, D. H.: Characteristics of the structural components of the mouse mammary tumor virus. 1. Morphological and biochemical studies. Virology **46**, 1 (1971).
35. Sarkar, N. H., Moore, D. H.: The internal structure of mouse mammary tumor virus as revealed after Tween-ether treatment. J. Micro. (Paris) **7**, 539 (1968).
36. Duesberg, P. H., Cardiff, R. D.: Structural relationships between the RNA of mammary tumor virus and those of other RNA tumor viruses. Virology **36**, 696 (1968).
37. Spiegelman, S., Burny, A., Das, M. R., Keydar, J., Schlom, J., Travnicek, M., Watson, K.: RNA-directed DNA polymerase activity in oncogenic RNA viruses. Nature (Lond.) **227**, 1029 (1970).
38. Temin, H. M., Mizutani, S.: RNA-dependent DNA polymerase in virions of Rous sarcoma virus. Nature (Lond.) **226**, 1211 (1970).
39. Baltimore, D.: RNA-dependent DNA polymerase in virions of RNA tumor viruses. Nature (Lond.) **226**, 1209 (1970).
40. Nowinski, R. C., Sarkar, N. H., Old, L. J., Moore, D. H., Scheer, D. J., Hilgers, J.: Characteristics of the structural components of the mouse mammary tumor virus. II. Viral proteins and antigens. Virology **46**, 21 (1971).
41. Blair, P. B.: Strain specificity in mouse mammary tumor virus virion antigens. Cancer Res. **31**, 1473 (1971).
42. Blair, P. B.: Immunology of the mouse mammary tumor virus (MTV): Neutralization of MTV by mouse antiserum. Cancer Res. **28**, 148 (1968).
43. Charney, J., Moore, D. H.: Immunization studies with MTV. J. nat. Cancer Inst. **48**, 1125 (1972).
44. Nowinski, R. C., Sarkar, N. H.: Serological and structural studies of mouse mammary tumor virus. J. nat. Cancer Inst. **48**, 1169 (1972).
45. Nowinski, R. C., Old, L. J., Sarkar, N. H., Moore, D. H.: Common properties of the oncogenic RNA viruses (oncornaviruses). Virology **42**, 1152 (1970).
46. Chopra, H. C., Mason, M. M.: A new virus in a spontaneous mammary tumor of a rhesus monkey. Cancer Res. **30**, 2081 (1970).
47. Nowinski, R. C., Edynak, E., Sarkar, N. H.: Serological and structural properties of Mason-Pfizer monkey virus isolated from the mammary tumor of a rhesus monkey. Proc nat. Acad. Sci. (Wash.) **68**, 1608 (1971).

48. SCHLOM, J., SPIEGELMAN, S.: DNA polymerase activities and nucleic acid components of virions isolated from a primate spontaneous mammary carcinoma. Proc. nat. Acad. Sci. (Wash.) 68, 1613 (1971).

49. CHOPRA, H. C., BOGDEN, A. E., ZELLJADT, I., JENSEN, E. M.: Virus particles in a transplantable rat mammary tumor of spontaneous origin. Europ. J. Cancer 6, 287 (1970).

50. AHMED, M., KOROL, W., LARSON, D., MOLNAR, H., SCHIDLOVSKY, G.: Transformation of rat mammary cell cultures by R-35 virus isolated from spontaneous rat mammary adenocarcinoma. J. nat. Cancer Inst. 48, 1077 (1972).

51. SCHIDLOVSKY, G., AHMED, M., SLATTERY, S., LOWRY, G.: Electron microscopy of cell transformation by R-35 rat virus and comparative morphology with other oncogenic viruses. J. nat. Cancer Inst. 48, 1067 (1972).

52. MOORE, D. H., SARKAR, N. H., KRAMARSKY, B., LASFARGUES, E. Y., CHARNEY, J.: Some aspects of the search for a human mammary tumor virus. Cancer (Philad.) 28, 1415 (1971).

53. FELLER, W. F., CHOPRA, H. C.: Virus-like particles in human milk. Cancer (Philad.) 28, 1425 (1971).

54. SEMAN, G., GALLAGER, H. S., LUKEMAN, J. M., DMOCHOWSKI, L.: Studies on the presence of particles resembling RNA virus particles in human breast tumors, pleural effusions, their tissue cultures, and milk. Cancer (Philad.) 28, 1431 (1971).

55. MOORE, D. H., SARKAR, N. H., KELLY, C. E., PILLSBURY, N., CHARNEY, J.: Type B particles in human milk. Tex. Rep. Biol. Med. 27, 4 (1969).

56. MOORE, D. H., CHARNEY, J., KRAMARSKY, B., LASFARGUES, E. Y., SARKAR, N. H., BRENNAN, M. J., BURROWS, J. H., SIRSAT, S. M., PAYMSTER, J. C., VAIDYA, A. B.: Search for a human breast cancer virus. Nature (Lond.) 229, 611 (1971).

57. SARKAR, N. H., MOORE, D. H.: On the possibility of a human breast cancer virus. Nature (Lond.) 236, 103 (1972).

58. SARKAR, N. H., MOORE, D. H.: Electron microscopy in mammary cancer research. J. nat. Cancer Inst. 48, 105, 1051 (1972).

59. SCHLOM, J., SPIEGELMAN, S., MOORE, D. H.: RNA-dependent DNA polymerase activity in virus-like particles isolated from human milk. Nature (Lond.) 231, 97 (1971).

60. SCHLOM, J., SPIEGELMAN, S., MOORE, D. H.: Detection of high-molecular-weight RNA in particles from human milk. Science 175, 542 (1972).

61. CHARNEY, J., MOORE, D. H.: Neutralization of murine mammary tumour virus by sera of women with breast cancer. Nature (Lond.) 229, 627 (1971).

62. AXEL, R., SCHLOM, J., SPIEGELMAN, S.: Presence in human breast cancer of RNA homologous to mouse mammary tumor virus RNA. Nature (Lond.) 235, 32 (1972).

Hormonal Induction of Breast Cancer

M. B. LIPSETT

Hormonal induction of breast cancer in man has not been established. There are insubstantial clues pointing to the hormonal environment as one of the many factors relevant to the genesis of breast cancer. Since perhaps only one-third of human breast cancers are endocrine-sensitive, it may be difficult to delineate endocrine influences in a subset of the population of women with breast cancer. Possible hormonal alterations may be produced by genetic or environmental effects. For example, the sensitivity of breast tissue to estrogen concentrations may vary for genetic reasons, or the total estrogenic stimulus could be altered by intake of plant estrogens. Minimal changes in estrogen secretion rates, duration of prolactin secretion, and availability of estrogen to the tissue are physiologic parameters that are difficult to quantify within the normal population. Yet small changes persistent over many years could produce significant cocarcinogenic effects.

The condition most often cited as evidence of hormonal induction is femaleness. The incidence of carcinoma of the breast in men is one percent of that in women. But this is insufficient proof of direct hormonal intervention. The mass of epithelial tissue in the breast may be 100 times greater in women than in men. Thus, purely on statistical grounds, the likelihood of cancer in these cells would be correspondingly greater in women.

There are several salient observations of the epidemiologist that support a role for the endocrine system in the induction of breast cancer. Cessation of ovarian function, equated properly with marked decrease in estrogen levels, is associated with a decreased risk of breast cancer [1]. A role for progesterone cannot be excluded in view of the data showing that experimental mammary carcinoma induction is affected by progesterone administration [2].

The relatively recent finding [3] that early pregnancy has a protective effect for the subsequent development of breast cancer has been interpreted as evidence that hormonal status has important consequences for the induction of human breast cancer. Chemical and biologic reasons why this hypothesis does not seem tenable are discussed below. But, *a priori*, it does not seem likely that a brief change in the hormonal milieu would be a decisive event since induction of breast cancer may require 10 to 20 years. An alternative hypothesis is that the early cell differentiation is the agent leading to protection. If this be so, it suggests that events leading to development of breast cancer begin early in life. DE WAARD [5] has suggested from epidemiologic considerations that only one type of breast cancer may be endocrine sensitive.

More specific proposals about hormonal influences on breast cancer induction in man derive from the broad base of experimental cancer in animals. The role of estrogens as cocarcinogens in the mouse and the rat are well-known examples of such data. Since estrogens are important in all mammals for growth and differentiation of the ductal tissue of the breast, the translation of effects in the rodent to man has been attempted. The difficulties in testing the hypothesis that higher estrogen concentrations are associated with a greater risk of development of breast cancer are formidable. Apart from the purely methodologic and epidemiologic considerations, there is the real possibility that such effects must be sought 10 to 20 years before the overt appearance of breast cancer.

Estriol, one of the metabolites of estradiol and estrone, at certain concentrations in the experimental animal acts as an anti-estrogen [6]. LEMON [7] proposed that variations in the risk for development of breast cancer may be inversely correlated with the excretion of estriol and presented data from several sources [8]. Similarly, it was suggested that the protective effect of early pregnancy was a result of the high estriol excretion [4]. These hypotheses were supported by the results of a recent biochemical-epidemiologic study showing a relatively higher estriol excretion in Japanese women than in North American women [9] consonant with the decreased incidence of breast cancer in the Japanese.

Unfortunately, these hypotheses have not taken into account certain basic chemical and biologic data. Estriol in the urine is conjugated and more importantly is derived from estrone and estradiol in blood. Thus, in normal women, estriol is the substance present in largest amount in urine but is the lowest of the three classical estrogens in blood. If changes in urinary estriol in normal women have predictive value, this must be because hepatic metabolism is different, since the changes do not reflect blood estriol concentrations.

The biologic data also bear on this hypothesis. Although plasma free estriol increases during pregnancy, estradiol increases even more [10]. The result of this is that the total biologic estrogenic stimulus to the woman is greater during pregnancy than at any other time. Thus, any potential anti-estrogenic effect of estriol cannot be detected, and the protective effects of early pregnancy cannot be ascribed to increased estriol concentration or excretion.

It is no longer possible to think of estrogen and stimulation of breast tissue without also considering the possible role of prolactin. Estrogens cause release of prolactin and secretion of prolactin has been correlated with growth of the endocrine-responsive, DMBA-induced, rat mammary carcinoma [11]. Again if prolactin is involved in the induction of breast cancer, epidemiologic studies will be necessary to demonstrate this. Plasma prolactin concentrations in man fluctuate widely depending on stress, emotion, and a number of unknown variables. Thus, one or two measurements will not give a true picture of prolactin secretion. The assessment of prolactin secretion and the subsequent comparison of population groups presents formidable obstacles.

Finally, it is necessary to relate the many reports of Bulbrook's group to the question of hormonal induction of cancer. Empirically, it was noted that the excretion of etiocholanolone, a 17-ketosteroid, had prognostic significance for the outcome of palliative procedures such as adrenalectomy and hypophysectomy. Since these data suggested that the steroid milieu was involved in tumor responsiveness, they subsequently tested the hypothesis that the steroid milieu was one factor in the induction of breast cancer. The most recent data from this prospective study [12] showed that etiocholanolone excretion was lower in women who developed breast cancer some years later than in matched normal controls. These are the only data from a prospective study that indicate that biochemical measurement has predictive value for risk of development of breast cancer.

It is not clear how to relate these findings to physiologic processes. Etiocholanolone in urine is derived principally from the metabolism of dehydroepiandrosterone, a steroid secreted by the adrenal cortex and without known biologic function. A lower excretion of etiocholanolone could indicate a lower secretion rate of its precursor, dehydroepiandrosterone, a lesser rate of metabolism of dehydroepiandrosterone to etiocholanolone, or a deviation of normal metabolic pathways. Intensive work will be needed to distinguish among these possibilities. Nevertheless, the observation, although not interpretable physiologically, is most important as a starting point for studies of the endocrine system and induction of breast cancer.

In summary, three decades of investigation into the relationships between breast cancer and hormones in man have yielded inconclusive results. From the data cited above and Jensen's recent reports (see chapter), there now appear to be substantial reasons for believing that the physician will be able to distinguish between those cancers that may be influenced by hormones and those that are not. Whether this ultimately reflects the genesis of the cancer or the hormonal milieu is work for the future.

References

1. Feinleib, M.: Breast cancer and artificial menopause. A cohort study. J. nat. Cancer Inst. 41, 315 (1968).
2. Muhlbock, O., Boot, L. M.: The mode of action of ovarian hormones in the induction of mammary cancer in mice. Biochem. Pharmacol. 16, 627 (1967).
3. MacMahon, B., Cole, P., Lin, T. M., Lowe, C. R., Mirra, A. P., Ravnihar, B., Salber, E. J., Valaoras, V. G., Yuasa, S.: Age at first birth and breast cancer risk. Bull. Wld Hlth Org. 43, 209 (1970).
4. Cole, P., MacMahon, B.: Oestrogen fractions during early reproductive life in the aetiology of breast cancer. Lancet 1969 I, 604.
5. de Waard, F.: The epidemiology of breast cancer; review and prospects. Inst. J. Cancer 4, 577 (1969).
6. Huggins, C., Jensen, E. V.: The depression of estrone-induced uterine growth by phenolic estrogens with oxygenated functions at positions 6 or 16; the impeded estrogens. J. exp. Med. 102, 335 (1955).
7. Lemon, H. M.: Endocrine influences on human mammary cancer. A critique. Cancer (Philad.) 23, 781 (1969).
8. Lemon, H. M., Wotiz, H. H., Parsons, L., Mozden, P. J.: Reduced estriol excretion in patients with breast cancer prior to endocrine therapy. J. Amer. med. Ass. 1961, 1128 (1966).
9. MacMahon, B., Cole, P., Brown, J. B., Aoki, K., Lin, T. M., Morgan, R. W., Woo, N. C.: Oestrogen profiles of Asian and North American women. Lancet 1971 II, 900.
10. Loriaux, D. L., Ruder, H. J., Knab, D. R., Lipsett, M. B.: Estrone sulfate, estrone, estradiol and estriol plasma levels in human pregnancy. J. clin. Endocr., in press.
11. Pearson, O. H., Molina, A., Butler, T. P., Llerena, L., Nasr, H.: Estrogens and prolactin in mammary cancer. In Estrogen, Target Tissues and Neoplasia. Ed.: T. L. Dao. Chicago: Univ. Chicago Press 1972.
12. Bulbrook, R. D., Hayward, J. L., Spicer, C. C.: Relation between urinary androgen and corticoid excretion and subsequent breast cancer. Lancet 1971 II, 395.

Appearance and Spread of Human Breast Cancer*

B. J. KENNEDY

Breast cancer is the most common form of cancer in females, comprising 23% of cancers in women and 13% of all cancers. The impact of this disease on the patient and her family can be devastating. Early detection of breast cancer can provide a curative approach to this disease; other forms of therapy can control the disease and provide the opportunity to prolong significant life. The study of the biologic behavior of breast cancer reveals the mode of appearance of early breast cancer and the nature of its spread.

The incidence of breast cancer is directly proportional to age. The older the patient, the greater the chance of developing breast cancer. It has been postulated that the process of aging and the process of developing a breast cancer may be comparable; that is, a decrease in the immunocompetence of the patient may result in deterioration of cell growth and the formation of a cancer. It is proposed that our immunologic system rejects cancers that may be formed daily, but as the process of aging proceeds and immunocompetence diminishes, cancer may form.

There is little idea of when a breast cancer begins and how long it takes to manifest itself clinically. At some point in time, a breast cancer does begin, enlarges, and eventually makes its clinical appearance. The principle of cancer detection is to establish the presence of the disease at as early a phase as possible. Improvements in cancer detection techniques make this a reality.

Early detection of breast cancer is aided by emphasizing the indices that lead to the possibilities for suspicion of an existing breast cancer. An increase in the incidence of breast cancer can be expected in unmarried, nulliparous women, those with a high familial incidence of breast cancer, and those with a previous history of benign breast disease. Certainly, a woman with one breast cancer has a greater risk for a new cancer in the opposite breast.

Techniques of breast examination are provided that allow us to determine the presence of this disease before it is apparent to the patient and even before it is clinically evident in the ordinary physical examination. These include mammography, thermography, xerography, transillumination, and cytology of nipple discharge. Although not practical for routine surveys, their use is warranted in patients who are at high risk for breast cancer or to reinforce the physician's clinical examination.

Optimal examination of a breast is carried out within the week after the menstrual period in premenopausal women, providing the least distraction from the

* This research was supported in party by grants CA-08101, CA-08832, and CA-05158 from the National Cancer Institute, United States Public Health Service.

physiological changes of the normal breast. A physician must be aware of these changes to aid him in the interpretation of nodularity of the normal breast and to recognize the difference between these changes and neoplastic alterations.

Clinically apparent disease can be described in terms of its earliest visibility and contiguous spread through the breast. A sequence of lesions can be described that illustrate the progressive nature of breast cancer.

1. Paget's disease of the nipple is an early superficial lesion. The prognosis of this disease is well established and with the lack of a palpable mass, simple mastectomy provides an adequate approach to cure. In the presence of palpable mass in the breast, conventional radical mastectomy is more appropriate.

2. Mammograms provide early detection of breast cancer before it is clinically apparent to an examiner. It is by this technique that the earliest manifestation of a tumor mass within the breast can be detected.

3. Skin retraction begins when the lesion enlarges sufficiently to alter the structure of Cooper's ligaments leading to various distortions of the overlying surface. Continuing enlargement of the mass leads to changes such as nipple eversion, nipple inversion, and more marked skin retraction.

4. As the lesion becomes more extensive in the breast, multiple retraction of the skin and/or lobularity of the breast are noted. By this time, the disease has extended sufficiently in size to render long term therapeutic results by mastectomy less effective.

It is a fact of life, however, that women will delay consulting a physician because of changes in the breast. Continued enlargement of the mass may occur before therapy is introduced; no longer are the benefits of early detection possible.

5. Replacement of the breast occurs as continued tumor growth progresses. Destruction of the breast ensues leading to a decrease in its size and ulceration. Satellite nodules appear on the skin. These changes characterize the nature of an enlarging breast mass that spreads in a contiguous manner.

6. Inflammatory carcinoma: Another manifestation of the appearance of breast cancer is that of a diffuse boggy breast with erythema and/or edema of the skin. This involvement of the subdermal lymphatics resembles an inflammatory process and is an inoperable situation. The disease quickly spreads to the opposite breast or to the shoulders and back. The prognosis is unusually poor.

The biological nature of breast cancer differs in regard to the appearance of the original tumor mass. By and large, breast cancer appears as involvement of the breast and because of this, early detection is a possibility. Only rarely does breast cancer appear initially as disseminated disease where the primary lesion is so small that it is undetectable by clinical examination. The primary tumor of breast cancer thus can appear as (I) an operable lesion, (II) a local lesion that is inoperable, and (III) disseminated disease with a very small mass undetectable by usual examination. It has been considered that the locally inoperable lesion and those situations with manifestations of disseminated disease as the first presenting findings reflect differences in the biologic behavior of these tumors [1]. Perhaps an immunologic system able to curtail the spread of cancer, confining it to the local area of the breast, may account for the differences in presentation. The cellular nature of the tumor itself differs also, and because of these differences, subsequent therapeutic results and prognosis vary considerably.

Role of the Contraceptive Pill in Breast Cancer

Previous studies have established that administration of small physiologic doses of estrogenic hormone to premenopausal women may result in stimulation of the growth of an existing breast cancer. If one extrapolates from the number of patients with disseminated disease that respond to bilateral ovariectomy, up to 40% of women who develop breast cancer in the premenopausal age group would be susceptible to stimulation of an existing breast cancer by administered estrogenic hormone. The contraceptive pills currently employed contain small amounts of estrogens, and therefore, can produce stimulation of hormone dependent tumors already existing in the breast. There is no data to suggest that the contraceptive pill causes human breast cancer. If existing breast cancers are stimulated by the contraceptive pill, in time there should appear a greater incidence of breast cancer in young women in the third decade. If the rate of growth is augmented, the lesion that may take several years to evolve clinically could be stimulated rapidly enough, manifesting itself earlier, and therefore, be detected at an earlier age.

The possibility of stimulation of an existing breast cancer in premenopausal women emphasizes the need for the physician to examine women in this age group receiving contraceptive medication at least three times a year. If a breast cancer is present and/or is stimulated by the estrogens, early detection of breast cancer would occur.

Two problems have arisen with respect to development of nodular breasts in women taking contraceptive medication: Frequently a history of having taken the contraceptive pill is not documented in records of patients with breast cancer. Many physicians assume that young women are receiving contraceptive pill therapy and fail to record this fact. Secondly, increased nodularity of the breast occurs during the use of the contra-contraceptive pill. This may be passed off as normal physiologic changes of the breast, rather than raising in the physician's mind a high index of suspicion of a breast cancer. Such a lesion can easily be advanced when finally recognized.

Early Detection of Breast Cancer

It is a common practice to classify patients with breast cancer by clinical stage on the basis of the clinical examination of the breast and axilla. Clinical Stage I disease is that limited to the breast without palpable axillary nodes. The presence of palpable nodes places a patient in Stage II. The existence of nodal metastases is a true determinent of a patient's prognosis.

Early detection of breast cancer provides a high rate of control in patients treated by mastectomy. At the University of Minnesota Cancer Detection Center, examinations have revealed that in patients whose lesions have been detected early and do not involve the axillary nodes, the observed five year survival is 97% and the 15 year survival is 87% [2]. With the presence of lymph nodes detected at the time of routine annual examination, the five year survival was 87.5% and the ten year survival, 57% [3]. It is of special interest to note that a relatively small group of patients with cancer found during the intervals between examinations had evidence of spread to lymph nodes or beyond, in spite of having had no recognizable cancer at the preceding examination. Survival for this group was extremely unfavorable (Table); so much so as to suggest that a basic biologic difference may exist between these "interval" patients and other patients seen at the Cancer Detection Center who developed breast cancer. This biologically different group may resemble those whose primary tumor is associated with distant dissemination of the disease.

Calculations of the relative survival rates of patients seen at the Cancer Detection Center demonstrate an extremely favorable result for patients whose cancers were without lymph node involvement at the time of surgery. When comparing survival of this group of patients with age corrected survival rates, the relative fifteen year

Table. Survival of patients with breast cancer at the University of Minnesota Cancer Detection Center [2, 3]

Observed survival	5 years	10 years	15 years
Negative lymph nodes	97%	91%	87%
Positive lymph nodes	87%	57%	66%
Positive lymph nodes (interval cases) [a]	45%	34%	11%

[a] See text.

survival (132%) was better than the normal population. Augmentation of survival appears to have occurred as the result of periodic follow-up attention to other concomitant health problems. Comparing these findings to standard figures of 69% fifteen year survival suggests that patients with breast cancers which were felt early had their life expectancy minimally jeopardized by the risk of dying from a cancer [2].

Recently a study of the correlation between clinical examination of the axillary lymph nodes and the histologic content of these nodes was made [4]. The study of 174 patients revealed that 55 patients had palpable axillary nodes, thus classifying them as Clinical Stage II. In Stage I, although the clinical examination revealed no lymphoadenopathy, 26% of the patients had histologic evidence of tumor. Furthermore, in 55% of the patients with clinically palpable disease, no lymph node metastases were noted in routine sections of the nodes. By only employing routine histologic sections, the possibility of missing disease is a reality. Thus, it appears that in women with cancer of the breast, palpable axillary nodes do not necessarily contain tumor; moreover, tumor deposits may be present in nodes which are not palpable. In the light of such knowledge of node histology, clinical status of nodes looses relevance to prognosis.

The Spread of Breast Cancer

The method of spread of breast cancer is threefold: via the axillary or internal mammary chains of lymph nodes, via subdermal lymphatics, or via the hematogenous route. Although even the smallest lesion may invade a vein wall, the larger the lesion, the greater the possibility of spread. Even then, tumor cells disseminated by a hematogenous route may not survive at the place of deposition.

Eventually, dissemination of the disease occurs. The disease may be manifest by a preponderance of metastases located in a single system, such as the bones, or in multiple combined areas such as the skin, lungs, and bones. The factors involved in the selection of sites of predilection are not understood. The nature of the metastases further demonstrate the biological differences in the characteristic of breast cancer. For example, a lung metastasis may be a single isolated nodule, or metastases may be multiple nodules or characterized by diffuse spread through the lymphatic channels. The latter are usually associated with a more severe prognosis than the discrete lesions. Furthermore, pleural effusion has a less severe prognosis than intrapulmonary lesions.

Studies of advanced breast cancer have attempted to define the clinical characteristics of the metastases by a staging procedure. The Cooperative Breast Cancer Group of the National Cancer Institute classified breast cancer according to the menopausal age and the dominant site of the metastases [5]. In that system, the site carrying the poorest prognosis was used as a basis for classification. *Breast and soft tissue* metastases, represented by the locally recurrent skin lesions and regional lymph nodes, have the best prognosis. *Osseous* metastases with or without soft tissue lesions were rated second in prognosis and *visceral* leisons, such as involvement of the liver, lung, and central nervous system with or without osseous and soft tissue lesions were regarded as having the poorest prognosis. These three dominant groups then were separated into four categories according to the number of years postmenopausal. This classification system provided an opportunity to compare clinical material between institutions. That study indicated that multiple site involvement could be handled simply. However, it is known that metastases in the lung and pleura have a more favorable prognosis than metastases in the liver and central nervous system. Hence, the visceral dominant site was too inclusive in their classification system. Although this system of classification was reasonable, a more descriptive method for summarizing the extent of the disease was considered to be more useful [6].

With more complete information on the history and clinical course of breast cancer patients involved in therapy trial studies, the results of cooperative studies could be more meaningful. A useful staging system of disseminated cancer has been developed utilizing the number of sites of dissemination of the cancer [6]. The designated sites were bone, lymph nodes, lung, skin, pleura, operative site, breast, and other areas. Of 920 patients, 111 patients had metastases in four sites which appeared to be associated with a high mortality. These sites were the liver, peritoneum, brain, or spinal cord. Patients with metastases to any one of these regions had a median survival of six months. This group was, therefore, termed the "dire prognosis" group and analyzed separately regardless of the number of sites of metastases involved.

The interval from diagnosis of the primary cancer in the breast to diagnosis of disseminated disease was found to be of profound prognostic significance. The longer the interval, the greater the survival time subsequent to diagnosis of disseminated disease. This corroborated a previous study [7]. Among patients with metastases in other than the "dire prognosis" sites, there was relatively little variation in survival with respect to specific sites of metastases. In contrast, there was marked variation in survival with respect to the number of sites involved. The more sites involved, the shorter the survival time.

Patients with distant metastases at the time of the initial diagnosis of breast cancer do not follow the same prognostic pattern as those with metastases arising following mastectomy. Those with the primary tumor and distant metastases should be analyzed

separately from the experience of women who develop disseminated disease subsequent to treatment of the primary cancer. That a biological difference in this group
appears to be present has been repeatedly recorded in the past.

As a result of this study, a classification system for disseminated breast cancer was
established. The number of sites of metastases were tabulated from 1 to 4, plus a fifth
"dire prognosis" group. This staging system, taking into consideration the effect of
the number of sites of metastases, offers a method of evaluation of disseminated breast
cancer for therapeutic trials and can be correlated with menopausal age as well.

It is quite clear that classification of disseminated breast cancer is required for
the careful evaluation of treatment results. Such studies are frequently conducted by
large institutions which may involve referral of the patients from community hospitals
or physicians. That the referral pattern changes and the type of patient admitted to
such study group changes, is now quite clear.

The Cooperative Breast Cancer Group, using the classification of the dominant
site methods, recorded an incidence of improvement of 22% in disseminated breast
cancer with testosterone propionate therapy in the first three years of a six year study
interval. The immediate following three years, the same group, using the same treatment method, recorded an incidence of 9.9% regression [8]. In an evaluation of the
explanation for this change, it became quite clear that one of the factors involved was
a decrease in the number of patients in the soft tissue breast dominant group, and an
increase in the number of patients entered into the visceral category. With this shift of
patients from a favorable group to an unfavorable group, the resulting decrease in the
regression rate could be explained. It is strikingly apparent that the evaluation of
chemotherapeutic results with advanced breast cancer strongly requires a randomized
ongoing study which takes into account the evaluation of the type of disease being
treated by the treatment group.

As investigators continue their work with disseminated breast cancer, it is inevit-
able that these groups face a change in the nature of disseminated disease. As medical
students and physicians are taught the conventional methods of therapy, these are
applied to the practicing physician's patients. Only when these standard therapies
fail to control the disease is the patient referred to an investigation group involving
newer methods of therapy. Hence, the research in advanced breast cancer is associated
with a changing population of disseminated disease due to the progress made in
previous years in the methods of control of the disease. That some investigators may
have access to clinical material of the same type they worked with 20 years before
even more strongly illustrates the need to classify the advanced disease so that data
between research groups and different institutions can be compared.

Conclusion

The study of breast cancer involves a range of problems from epidemiology, early
appearance, early detection, management of the primary disease, management of the
recurrent and disseminated disease, treatment of the patient in the supportive phase
of the disease where antitumor therapies are not effective, and treatment of the
patient during the dying phase of the disease. The biological nature of breast cancer is
variable. The factors involved include the chronological age of the patient, the menopausal age, the interval between the primary treatment and the dissemination of the

disease, and the sites of metastases. Indeed the nature of the appearance of breast cancer and its mode of spread is a science unto itself and is closely allied with the therapeutic potentials and survival of the patient. With a clear understanding of the biological nature of breast cancer, the physician can contribute significantly to the possible cure and control of breast cancer.

References

1. KENNEDY, B. J.: Hormone therapy in inoperable breast cancer. Cancer (Philad.) 24, 1345 (1969).
2. GILBERTSEN, V. A., KJELSBERG, M.: Detection of breast cancer by periodic utilization of methods of physical diagnosis. Cancer (Philad.) 28, 1552 (1971).
3. GILBERTSEN, V. A.: Personal communications.
4. WALLACE, I. W. J., CHAMPION, H. R.: Axillary nodes in breast cancer. Lancet 1972 I, 217.
5. Cooperative Breast Cancer Group: Progress Report: Results of studies by the Cooperative Breast Cancer Group — 1956—60. Cancer Chemother. Abstr. 11, 109 (1961).
6. CUTLER, S. J., ASIVE, A. J., TAYLOR, III, S. G.: Classification of patients with disseminated cancer of the breast. Cancer (Philad.) 24, 861 (1969).
7. Council on Drugs, Subcommittee on Breast and Genital Cancer: Androgens and estrogens in the treatment of disseminated mammary carcinoma: Retrospective study of nine hundred forty-four patients. J. Amer. med. Ass. 188, 1069 (1964).
8. Cooperative Breast Cancer Group: Results of studies of the Cooperative Breast Cancer Group, 1961—1963. Cancer Chemother. Abstr. 41 (Suppl. 1), 1—24 (1964).

Early Detection of Breast Cancer: X-Ray, Ultrasound, Thermography

R. L. EGAN

There are many roles of mammography in the detection, diagnosis, treatment planning, and prognosis of breast cancer. The three primary areas are:

1. stimulation of interest in the disease by medical profession;
2. appeal to the patient and hope that a cure might result; and
3. provision of earlier and more comprehensive treatment of the patient with breast cancer.

The stable incidence, survival and mortality rates in breast cancer suggest a major reorientation may be indicated in the concept of the origin, pathogenesis, natural history and management of cancer of the breast. Three-fourths of a century has passed since Halstead reported on the results of his radical operation for carcinoma of the breast. Mammography has been labeled as the procedure that has done more for the breast cancer patient since his report at the turn of the century. To my knowledge no medical procedure has been tested and retested as much as mammography.

In 1956 the introduction of an adequate, safe, simple, accurate and reproducible radiographic technique of breast examination coincided with a controversial period in the history of breast cancer. It was the most feared cancer, a cancer treated most radically, the cancer that involved the most surgical operations the most radiation therapy, the most chemotherapy, the most hormone therapy, and was the most costly cancer in dollars. Despite a very high incidence of the disease there has been a very low salvage rate.

The breasts were most accessible to clinical examination. Women were delaying seeking medical care due to fear and lack of rapport with the physicians yet physicians were missing 25% of these relatively advanced cancers on initial examination. There was no satisfactory classification of breast diseases by the pathologists and there was no uniformity in definitive or palliative treatment. Lack of knowledge of the natural history of breast cancer persisted even though it had been recognized for centuries and had provoked much controversy. There was a minimum of rapport between the patient, the referring physician, the surgeon, the radiologist and the pathologist despite intimate involvement of each specialty with this disease.

Mammography is our only reliable means of detecting breast cancer prior to signs and symptoms. This aspect has created interest in other approaches to earlier detection of breast cancer, such as ultrasound, xeroradiography, isotope scanning and thermography and then mammography acts as a thoroughly investigated yardstick to gauge the value of these procedures. At present all these procedures have not had the extensive proven application of mammography and, until such time, may be regarded as laboratory procedures with great ancillary potential.

Mammography establishes a rapport between the physician and the patient; the patient feels that something special is being done for her. This use, in fact, is immeasurable and might be quite significant since the patients still find 95% of their breast cancers. Mammography then prevents delay in instituting treatment of breast cancers.

Mammography is our best means of differentiating the second primary breast cancer from metastatic disease. Proper detection and treatment of the second breast cancer alone would increase the ten year salvage rate by an estimated 150%.

Mammography affords the recognition of almost ten times as many bilateral simultaneous primary cancers when compared with routine detection methods.

Mammography is providing entirely new stages of breast cancers by demonstrating cancers that cannot be palpated.

There is conclusive evidence that by mammography many breast cancers can be detected as long as two years prior to clinical recognition. This suggests a potential use of mammography in screening of the general population for breast cancer. However at present, the use of mammography is used in patients in high-risk groups, not as a routine survey screening test. This application is being investigated.

Mammography has proved to be our best means of studying the natural history of breast diseases. Prior to mammography, rarely was the term pre-malignant disease of the breast used. The team approach to study breast cancer has centered around mammography and has led to correlated clinical, radiologic and pathologic whole organ studies of the breast. Minute detail on the mammograms of specimen radiographs can be compared with histopathologic preparations. Certain changes are merely variants of normal, but, in a rather orderly manner there is a progression from proliferative epithelial hyperplasia, that includes papillomatosis, to metaplasia and anaplasia of these cells to carcinoma in-situ, and finally to frank invasive carcinoma of the breast. Eventually, such continued studies should lead to recognition of that pre-malignant stage of irreversibility signalling prompt patient treatment.

A problem so enormous as carcinoma of the breast can easily be shared by a team of general practitioner, surgeon, radiologist and pathologist. The best applications of mammography are obtained by the radiologist who realizes the limitations of the procedure, the pathologist who strives conscientiously at all times to study the proper tissue, and the surgeon and radiotherapist that combine the findings of their colleagues with their own clinical judgment.

Mammography has forced the radiologist, surgeon and pathologist to work closely together to detect breast cancer at an earlier stage, to institute more comprehensive treatment and to effect a lowering of the mortality from breast cancer.

At Emory University Hospital, operating in a community where rapport has been established with potential breast cancer patients and where the interdisciplinary approach is active, 80% of the operable patients have Stage 0 or Stage I breast cancer. In the 10% of our patients with clinically unsuspected breast cancers, 92% have the axilla free of metastatic disease. If the lesion must be localized by radiography of the biopsy specimen for the pathologist, nearly 100% have negative axillary lymph nodes. In this latter group, the cancer may not be palpated in 3 mm thick sections after localization by radiography for the pathologist.

There is no question that use of mammography will have real impact on treatment and prognosis of breast cancer. The knowledge that breast cancer can be cured will become disseminated in more and more communities.

If this experience were extended to thousands of American communities a real impact could occur on breast cancer mortality.

Cancer of the breast is a dread disease and, by its very nature, has a severe psychological effect on its victims. Seemingly intelligent women still present themselves with "advanced" cancer of the breast; the history is often one of having been observed for a variable period of time by a physician or the patient having been reluctant to submit to early examinations fearing that the correct diagnosis could not be reached short of mutilation. Some other approach is required to educate American women. A simple, inexpensive, nontraumatic, reliable procedure for the diagnosis of the breast lesions could remove the apprehension of this disease, hospital bills, indecision and loss of time.

An immeasurable psychologic impact is also occurring in many communities. Less aggresive surgery is required with the cancer limited to the breast. There is still need for radical removal of the breast but less radical surgery of the axilla and pectoral muscles [1]. Formerly each woman with a breast lump envisioned results of her proposed surgery to equal edema of the arm, the worst scarring of the chest wall, and limitation of motion of the arm as she has seen in other patients. Women cured of breast cancer with no edema of the arm and completely normal activity and appearance will convince other women treatment of the breast lump is neither fatal nor mutilating.

Now that earlier breast cancer has been detected by mammography, what does it mean? Patients with the smallest cancer and the less metastasis to the lymph nodes still have the most favorable prognosis. At Emory, breast cancer patients without axillary lymph node metastasis had a 70% 10-year salvage as compared to 29% survivors with positive axillary nodes—an impressive difference indicating the value of the team approach to breast cancer.

It seems appropriate to reemphasize the conclusions reached by GALLAGER [1] and seven other authorities in the recent panel discussion at the Ninth Annual Mammography Seminar:

"Only a dozen years ago, the management of breast cancer was 'cut and dried' affair. A women found a lump in her breast, reported it to her physician, a biopsy of the mass was done with frozen section and, if carcinoma was found, radical mastectomy followed. An early cancer meant a barely palpable mass without the slightest attachment to skin or underlying structures, and was only a little less likely to have produced axillary spread then a tumor obvious to the examiner's fingers.

Today, this attitude is in the process of rapid change. Thanks largely to mammography, we are able to detect a malignant breast neoplasm long before it forms a mass. Because we know that cure rates in this stage are high, we are deeply concerned

---

1 We still do radical or "complete" mastectomies.

with reliable means of early detection and diagnosis. Early detection has certainly been the major influence in reduction of mortality from cancer of the cervix and the results of recent studies indicates that this will also be true for the breast."

Reference

1. GALLAGER, H. S., FARROW, J. H., GALANTE, M., GRAY, L. A., MARTIN, J. R., OZELLA, L., TAYLOR, H. B., TAYLOR, W. J.: Early breast cancer: what is it. Sth. Med. Bull. 59, 10—12 (1971).

Recent Contributions to Our Knowledge about the Pathology of Breast Cancer

D. G. SCARPELLI and T. M. MURAD

Much of our knowledge concerning the pathology of breast cancer in humans has been gained from the study of this disease by the methods of classical morphology. This has resulted in a wealth of information on the various histologic types of malignant neoplasms of breast, their patterns of growth and modes of spread, and finally their prognosis based on careful and extensive correlative clinicopathologic studies. Despite these many advances it is clear that our knowledge of this disease is still far from complete. Recent studies employing the tools of classical morphology and those which extend its limits, such as electron microscopy, cytochemistry and immunochemistry, have added new knowledge and in certain instances challenged some of the old. The purpose of this communication will be to review some of the contributions made during the past five years as seen from the perspective of a general pathologist.

Clinicopathologic Studies

The clinicopathologic approach to the study of breast cancer continues to be one of the most pragmatically significant and productive, since it is based on the correlation of the morphologic alterations and patterns of the various types of neoplasms with their biological behavior. Single tumor cells arranged in tandem to form a column termed "single filing" is a peculiar histogenetic pattern which has drawn the attention of pathologists since the mid-nineteenth century and which has been variously interpreted as indicating that the neoplasm has a limited potential for malignant growth or conversely that it is highly malignant. Surprisingly, prior to the study of RICHTER et al. [1] of a large series of cases, no systematic clinicopathologic assessment of the biologic significance of this morphologic feature existed. According to these authors, single filing per se appeared to have no prognostic significance; the chances for survival in their series were similar to those of any patient with carcinoma of the breast. Prognosis in cases with the single filing pattern depended on the presence or absence of lymph node involvement and the length of time that had elapsed after mastectomy. The five-year survival of patients with the single filing phenomenon without lymph node involvement was 91.7% as compared to 82% for those with cancer of the breast of all histologic grades. On the other hand, the 10-year survival of patients with this histogenetic pattern with lymph node metastasis was only 9.3% as compared to 23.2% for those with grade 4 or anaplastic carcinoma, or 27.6% for those with cancer of all grades. This variable biological behavior in patients with and without positive lymph nodes makes single filing an unreliable morphologic feature upon which to base prognosis. The situation in breast cancer is in direct contrast to the uniformly poor prognosis encountered for carcinomas with this histogenetic pattern arising in stomach and colon where survival is much shorter than in the more common well differentiated adenocarcinomas of these organs.

In a somewhat different vein TAYLOR and NORRIS [2] reported a study of 33 cases of an infrequently encountered histogenetic variant of ductal carcinoma so well differentiated that eight of the cases in their series had been initially diagnosed as sclerosing adenosis. Although the primary tumors tended to be small in size, metastases to axillary lymph nodes were present in 30% of the cases. Despite this apparently aggressive biological behavior the prognosis appears to be quite favorable since nodal involvement is almost always limited to 1 or 2 nodes and death due to metastatic disease occurred in only one patient of the 33 studied. Well differentiated ductal carcinoma can appear so benign histologically that the authors describe it as "beguilingly innocuous". According to them it can be distinguished from sclerosing adenosis by virtue of its completely disorganized arrangement of neoplastic ducts, infiltrative growth pattern, loose reactive appearing stroma which accompanies the lesion, neoplastic ducts lined by a single layer of cells and finally the presence of intraductal carcinoma in about 60% of the lesions.

Attempts to improve the prognostication of breast cancer by virtue of an accurate assessment of histopathologic type continue to occupy the attention of pathologists, this in spite of the fact that clinicians seem to rely more heavily on the clinical staging of the disease rather than its histopathologic classification. CHRISTOPHERSON [3] emphasizes the need for employing the classification of FOOTE and STEWART [4] now the official classification of the World Health Organization [5], if the prognostic comparison of various series of cases of similar clinical stage is to be valid. This is so because, for similar stages of disease, variations in biological behavior from tumor to tumor are most probably due to variability in 1) the growth characteristics exhibited by the particular histogenetic variant, and 2) the complex of factors that constitute the host-tumor relationship. According to CHRISTOPHERSON [3] a large series of breast cancer cases under long term study at Memorial Cancer Center [6] shows that a relationship exists between the histopathologic type of carcinoma and patient survival; these relationships are summarized in the Table. The prognostic significance of the size of the breast tumor and the extent of axillary lymph node involvement are also pointed out in this communication [3].

A cytologic approach to prognostication of breast cancer has been reported by HARTVEIT [7] in a series of 222 cases in which a correlation was shown between certain cytologic characteristics of the tumor cells and patient survival. The results of this study indicated that tumors composed of cells characterized by irregularly shaped and lobulated (vacuolated) nuclei, and having scant cytoplasm and well-defined cell borders had the poorest prognosis with a survival of 7% (5 years) and 0% (10 years). In contrast tumors consisting of nonvacuolated, regular shaped nuclei with ample cytoplasm and well-defined borders had survival rates of 100% (5 years) and 69% (10 years). Although the criteria employed in this prognostic method include the well established cytologic characteristics for the diagnosis of malignancy, such as anisocytosis and a high nucleocytoplasmic ratio, nuclear vacuolization, and ill-defined cell borders are alterations which can occur as a consequence of cell injury, autolysis and poor fixation. It would seem more prudent to employ more rigorously controlled methods of tissue fixation utilizing 2—3 mm slices of freshly excised tissue and more efficient fixatives such as paraformaldehyde or glutaraldehyde, thus ensuring a minimum of cytologic artifacts. Future reports of similar studies will be awaited with great interest.

Table. Relationship between morphologic type of breast cancer, lymph node involvement and patient survival [a]

Type	% with nodal involvement	% Survival	
		5 years	10 years
Duct with productive fibrosis	60	54	38
Lobular	60	50	32
Comedo	32	73	58
Medullary	44	63	50
Colloid	32	73	59
Papillary	17	83	56

[a] Composite from CHRISTOPHERSON [3] after McDIVITT, STEWART, and BERG [6].

Efforts continue to be expended toward the morphologic diagnosis of breast cancer at a very early stage of the disease, indeed even at the presymptomatic stage. Although, there have not been major breakthroughs in this area of endeavor, there are several interesting studies which merit mention. POTTER et al. [8] carried out a follow-up study of women having had a previous benign breast lesion. The most significant finding in the 110 women who were successfully followed-up was that the occurrence rate of breast cancer was 480% higher than that of women of similar age from the general population. Another point of interest is that in this high risk group carcinoma developed in either the breast with the original benign lesion or the contralateral one 16 to 20 years after the initial biopsy. The greatest number of carcinomas occurred in the group of patients in which the original lesion had been a benign fibroadenoma. The next greatest incidence occurred in those groups of women with either an initial diagnosis of mammary dysplasia with sclerosing adenosis and epithelial hyperplasia, or in which the initial biopsy showed essentially normal or minimally inflamed breast tissue. This rather surprising finding not only emphasizes our ignorance about the long term biological significance of mammary dysplasia, but also highlights the limited sampling afforded by the biopsy. Continued long term clinical follow-up of the high risk group of women selected as a consequence of having suffered from a benign breast lesion certainly seems warranted. We have much to learn about the relationship between a benign lesion indicative of a biologically "restless" breast and subsequent development of carcinoma.

Methods for the presymptomatic diagnosis of breast cancer continue to be a major thrust of many workers [9]. Mammography, xerography and thermography are physical methods which offer great promise as potent tools for the early diagnosis of clinically inconspicuous malignant lesions of the breast. Studies by BULBROOK et al. [10] indicate that many patients with early breast cancer excrete lower than normal amounts of aetiocholanolone, an androgen metabolite, and higher than normal levels of 17-hydroxycorticosteroids in their urine. It is of interest to note that women who show this abnormal pattern of steroid excretion have a high recurrence and death rate. Whether these alterations exist during the initial pathogenesis of breast cancer remains to be seen; if they are, then this could serve as a means of isolating a high risk population of women which could be followed closely so therapeutic intervention could be accomplished at the first evidence that the neoplastic transformation had occurred. A morphologic approach to early diagnosis has been reported by STANLEY et al. [11] in which anomalies of the sex chromatin appears to exist in the buccal epithelium of women with breast cancer. Again it must be determined whether these alterations precede or follow the development of cancer. If it proves to be the former, this would be a simple, rapid and potent approach to the early diagnosis of mammary cancer.

In recent years more studies appear to be directed toward elucidating the nature and significance of host defense against tumor invasion and metastases of breast cancer. This is no doubt due in part to the recent promising developments in tumor immunology research. The morphologic aspects of the host defense reaction in patients with breast cancer have been the center of considerable controversy since the initial reports of BLACK et al. [12] in 1953. It is worthy of note that despite some rather withering attacks the question of the prognostic significance of sinus histiocytic proliferation in axillary lymph nodes draining breast cancer has been revived, and a number of other interesting observations dealing with the host defense reaction(s) have been reported. ANASTASSIADES and PRYCE [13] found that hyperplasia of the reticuloendothelial cells of the nodal sinuses and lymphocytes of lymph nodes in cases of breast cancer were associated with a low tendency for metastasis. This was especially so when the lymph node reaction was accompanied by a chronic inflammatory reaction in the tumor. In this series the overall rate of metastases for cases with sinus histiocytosis was 33% as contrasted to 68% in cases in which the reaction was absent. This differential in metastatic rate was also evident when the cases were separated and classified by their respective histopathologic grades. Thus, it appears that a favorable host reaction is manifest regardless of the degree of anaplasia exhibited by the neoplasm. According to these authors, certain cases showed lymph nodes which were hypocellular and markedly hyalinized, retrogressive changes suggestive of exhaustion of an immune response. They further point out that these cases like those in which there was no sinus reaction were characterized by a high rate of tumor metastasis. Essentially similar findings were reported by HAMLIN [14] and more recently BRIGHTMORE et al. [15], although in these studies emphasis was placed on the inflammatory reaction present within the tumor and at its periphery. The inflammatory reaction within the tumor along with the lymph node reaction is termed by these workers as the "host defense reaction". The former reaction is characterized by varying degrees of lymphocytic and plasma cell infiltration. In some instances these may include structures resembling germinal centers and pyroninophilic cells resembling "immunoblasts". These authors emphasize that a combination of factors appears to be involved in determining the prognosis of any given case of breast cancer;

these include, the delay period, clinical stage, size of tumor, histological characteristics of the tumor and the host defense reaction to it, and finally the absence or presence of axillary lymph node metastases. They also conclude that the nature and intensity of the inflammatory reaction within and around the tumor is of considerable biological importance, a view which corroborates and extends the earlier observations of Berg [16]. On the other hand, studies by Kister et al. [17] and Sommers [18] indicate that neither sinus histiocytosis nor inflammatory infiltrate within and around the tumor appears to be related to the biological behavior of breast cancers.

The foregoing reports on the morphologic components termed the host defense reaction(s) in breast cancer and their prognostic significance indicate that much remains to be learned. The increased numbers of reports of a correlation between the nature and intensity of these tissue reactions and the biological behavior of the tumor do not permit us to dismiss this approach out of hand. In view of the demonstration of tumor specific antigens in a variety of neoplasms and of impaired cell mediated immunity in cancer patients, continued study of these morphologic reactions seems warranted.

Kister et al. [17] also found no correlation between the degree of nuclear differentiation of tumor cells and their behavior. Sommers' [18] data, however, suggests that nuclear grading as proposed by Black and Speer [19] may be of prognostic value since well differentiated intraductal carcinomas consisted of neoplastic cells with differentiated nuclei as contrasted to the poorly differentiated nuclei present in undifferentiated invasive carcinomas. Continued careful studies of the relation of nuclear differentiation to tumor behavior will eventually place the significance of nuclear morphology in true perspective.

Despite the fact that the nature of the etiologic factor or factors responsible for the genesis of breast cancer in humans is still obscure, there is sufficient evidence to implicate disturbed hormonal relationships and endocrine imbalance as one of the factors. Since the breast is exquisitely sensitive to estrogenic hormones and responds to them by augmented growth, it is reasonable to expect studies directed toward elucidating the possible relationship between estrogenic hormones and breast cancer, especially with the widespread use of oral contraceptives.

A provocative and authoritative review by Lemon [20] points out the interrelation of C18 and C19 steroid metabolism to fibrocystic disease and carcinoma of the female breast. Within the C18 series of steroids, estriol has the unique effect of both competitively inhibiting the growth stimulatory effects of estradiol and displacing it from receptor proteins of the target cell. He postulates that a relative deficiency of estriol may allow for the stimulatory effects of estradiol to act unopposed on breast tissue with sufficient intensity and duration to be an important etiologic factor in human breast cancer. This view of disturbed hormone homeostasis is in keeping with the emerging data on the complex metabolic interrelationships which exist between the various estrogenic hormones and their biological significance.

Attempts to demonstrate enhanced binding of steroid hormones by breast cancer tissue have met with limited success, but the results have been sufficiently promising to warrant further studies along this line. Braunsberg et al. [21] have shown that following in vivo infusion of tritium (^{3}H) labeled estradiol malignant breast tumor tissue contained significantly higher concentrations of free steroid than did any other tissue studied including normal breast tissue, muscle, skin and adipose tissue. Testosterone-1,2-³H on the other hand did not show such striking concentration differences between malignant breast tumor and normal tissues. QUINCEY and GRAY [22] found no enhanced uptake of orally administered ³H-methyltestosterone by breast cancer tissue. It may be that these differences are due to the route of labeled hormone administration.

According to FECHNER [23] breast cancer which developed in women less than 35 years of age that were on a regular regimen of oral contraceptives was morphologically identical to that in women of similar age who had never used such hormone therapy, a finding counter to an earlier report by GOLDENBERG et al. [24]. Furthermore, FECHNER [23] states that in his series of cases the incidence of breast cancer in women under 35 years of age remains at about 4⁰/o of all breast cancers, a figure identical to that of other series studied prior to the advent of potent antiovulant compounds. Although this data is interesting, it is based on a rather limited number of cases; thus, the final answer must await a massive long term statistical study involving many thousands of women that have been regular users of oral contraceptives. The report of SYMMERS [25] of the development of metastasizing carcinoma of the breast in 2 transsexual individuals who had been on continuous and prolonged administration of estrogens, though admittedly a very limited series, emphasizes the possible role of estrogenic hormones in the pathogenesis of breast cancer.

As an added reminder that other hormonal factors may be operative in the genesis of breast cancer, the findings of CHALESTREY and BENJAMIN [26] of a high incidence of breast cancer in patients with carcinoma of thyroid treated by thyroidectomy merit mention. Presumably this relationship might be explained on the basis of excessive and prolonged stimulation of pituitary function as a consequence of a surgically induced hypothyroidism. This report fits well with an earlier one by HUMPHREY and SWERDLOW [27] in which it was shown that the incidence of breast cancer is considerably higher in women with thyroid disease than in the general female population.

Histogenesis and Classification of Breast Cancer

An understanding of the histogenesis of breast cancer must be based on a detailed knowledge of the embryology and cytology of the normal mammary secretory unit. The secretory unit develops from differentiation of ectodermal epithelium along the ventrolateral body wall, the so-called "milk lines" extending bilaterally from the axilla to the inguinal region. The ectoderm buds downward into the underlying connective tissue stroma and during the 4th month of fetal life the buds extend in various directions. The main buds form the major ducts; these then progressively branch and rebranch to form the smaller ducts (ductules) and finally the secretory acini. Formation of ducts, ductules and acini occurs by reconstruction of the solid cords of epithelium. Essentially this process consists of the progressive removal of cells to form an elongated hollow tube lined by cells, the blind end forming the acinus. It should be pointed out that in the breast as in other organs, the stroma plays an important role in the formation of the secretory unit. In fact, the relation is so intimate that the distinction between stromal and epithelial cell becomes blurred as evidenced by the still unclear origin of the myoepithelial cell. Some consider it as a modified epithelial cell originating from epithelium while others feel it is derived from the mesenchyme. The fully-differentiated secretory unit of the breast consists of ducts which branch into smaller ductules which in turn collect secretions extruded into the lumen of the individual alveoli which form the acini. Ultrastructural studies have shown that the duct consists of cuboidal cells containing short arrays of rough-surfaced endoplasmic reticulum, ovoid and short rod shaped mitochondria, and their apical surface consisting of short microvilli. These cells rest on a layer of myo-

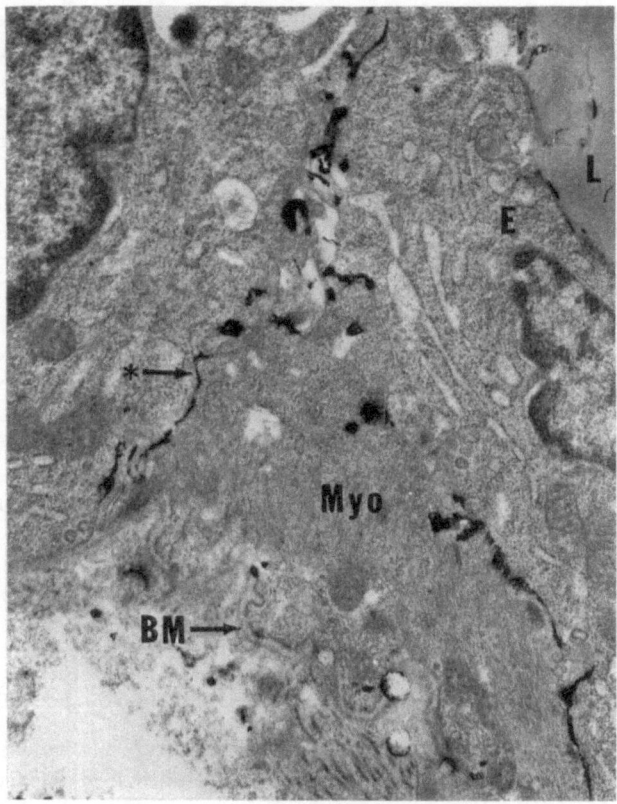

Fig. 1. Normal breast duct: ATP-ase activity is localized to the plasma membrane of a myoepithelial cell (Myo) which rests on the basement membrane (BM). An epithelial cell (E) lines the lumen (L) which contains dense amorphous secretory material. (×15,000)

epithelial cells which in turn abut on a basement membrane. The duct lumen is almost invariably fully patent; the degree of branching of the duct appears to depend on the degree of estrogen stimulation. The duct branches into ductules which in contrast to the former have no recognizable lumen. These are lined by cuboidal epithelium containing polysomal aggregates and large ovoid mitochondria. These cells are surrounded by an interlacing rather than a continuous layer of myoepithelial cells as is present in those lining the ducts. Since ductules are encountered only in female breasts they are very probably a developmental reflection of the hormonal milieu peculiar to them.

Cytochemical studies of "normal" human breast have shown that the localization of certain phosphatase enzymes varies among the three cell types that basically constitute the secretory unit. These localizations are sufficiently reproducible in these cells to serve as an identifying enzyme marker for them as shown by MURAD et al. [28]. The cytoplasm of duct and ductular epithelium has a weakly positive acid phosphatase activity which is reflected ultrastructurally by the presence of few lyso-

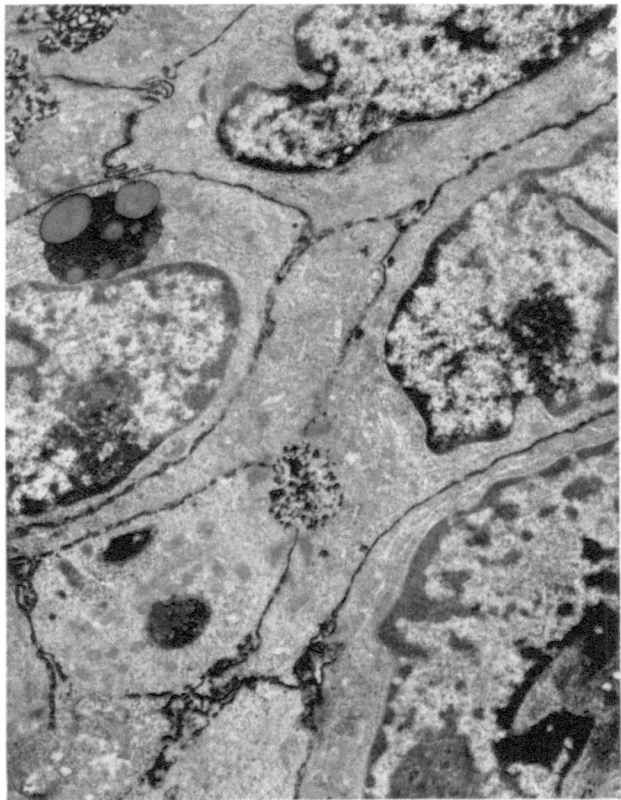

Fig. 2. Ductal carcinoma, myoepithelial variant: An intense ATP-ase reaction is localized on the plasma membrane of neoplastic myoepithelial cells. (×6,000)

somes. Both cell types have a very weak to absent adenosine triphosphatase (ATP-ase) activity on their plasma membranes and are devoid of alkaline phosphatase activity. On the other hand the myoepithelial cell has intense ATP-ase, inosine diphosphatase, (IDP-ase), and alkaline phosphatase activity localized on the plasma membrane (Fig. 1). Acid phosphatase is uniformly absent from myoepithelial cells as are lysosomal profiles in the cytoplasm.

The histogenesis of mammary carcinoma as reconstructed from systematic ultrastructural and cytochemical studies by MURAD [29, 30] suggests that these neoplasms can arise from any of the 3 cell types that constitute the breast secretory unit.

Neoplasms classified as ductal carcinomas by light microscopy could be subclassified on the basis of more careful study into two distinct groups. The first group consisted of neoplasms in which the tumor cells exhibited an intense ATP-ase and IDP-ase activity in the plasma membrane (Fig. 2), and a dense cytoplasm which contained occasional patches of fibrils (Fig. 3). These characteristics are so similar to those of the normal myoepithelium to suggest this as the cell of origin for this group of tumors.

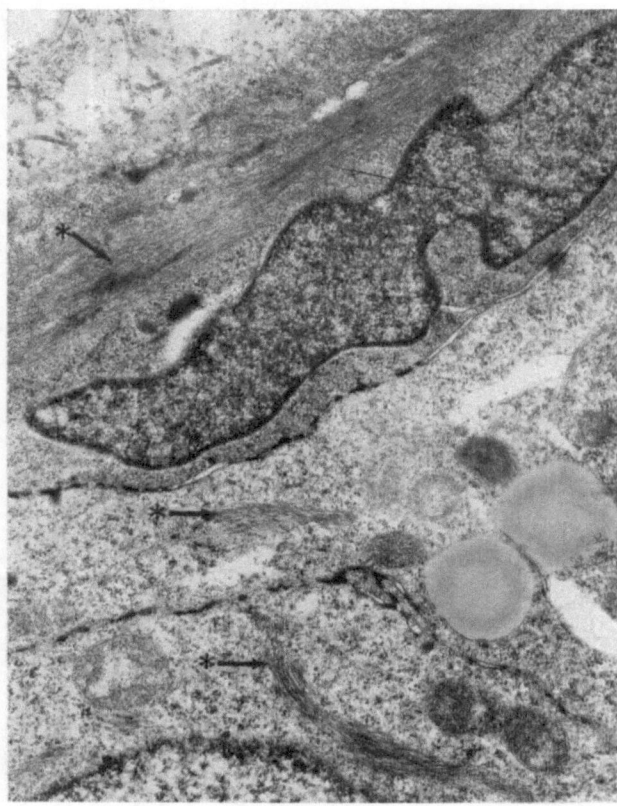

Fig. 3. Ductal carcinoma *in situ*, myoepithelial variant: Arrays of cytoplasmic fibrils resembling myofibrils (∗ →) are present in malignant myoepithelial cells. (×18,300)

The role of myoepithelial cells in carcinoma of the breast has been ably reviewed by HAMPERL [31].

The second group consisted of neoplasms in which the tumor cells were devoid of plasmalemmal ATP-ase and IDP-ase as demonstrated cytochemically. The cytoplasm contained a moderately well developed rough surfaced endoplasmic reticulum and moderate numbers of lysosomes in which acid phosphatase activity was demonstrated (Fig. 4), characteristics which suggest that these neoplasms were derived from ductal epithelium. Neoplasms arising from ductular epithelium could be differentiated from the other two by virtue of distinct cytologic and cytochemical characteristics. Tumor cells contained a well-developed rough surfaced endoplasmic reticulum and exhibited an acid phosphatase activity which in contrast to that in ductal carcinoma cells was diffusely distributed in the cytoplasm (Fig. 5). In addition, there was a curious localization of acid phosphatase in the heterochromatin of the nucleus. Abolition of this localization by heating of the tissues to 70° C for 15 min. prior to the cyto-chemical reaction suggests that it is due to enzymatic activity rather than diffusion or

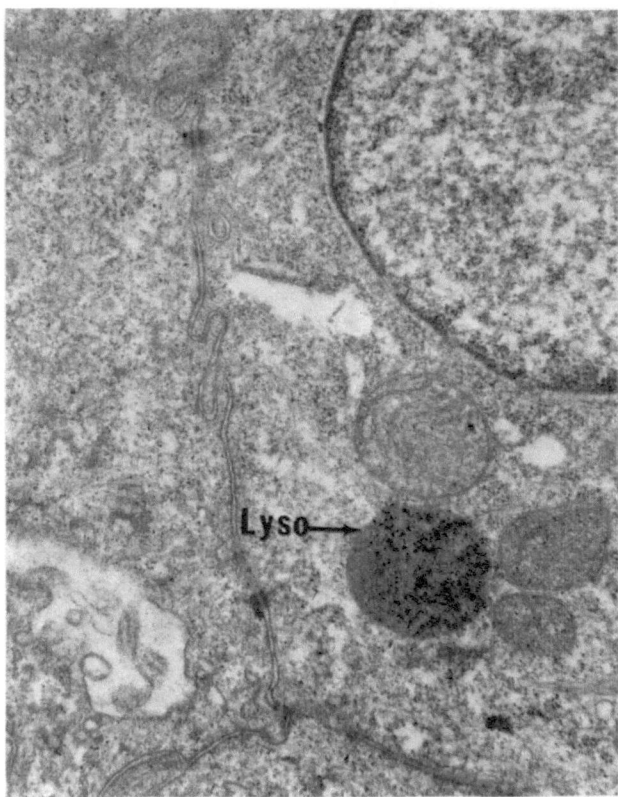

Fig. 4. Ductal carcinoma epithelial cell variant: Acid phosphatase activity localized in a lysosome (Lyso). (×21,300)

spurious binding. The plasma membrane was devoid of activity for any of the phos-phatase enzymes.

This classification, based on what appears to be distinct cytochemical differences between the various types of breast cancer cells, should be substantiated by the application of more precise biochemical methods. A promising approach would be to study the enzymatic profile of pure fractions of tumor cells isolated from stromal and other cells which comprise breast cancers by means of recently developed techniques involving zonal gradient centrifugation [32, 33]. Classification of breast cancer according to the cell of origin identifies the segment or segments of the breast secretory unit from which the neoplasm arose which may allow for a more rational approach to therapy, since the various segments differ in their response to certain chemicals and hormones. It would be of interest to ascertain if a relation existed between the cell of origin of a neoplasm and its degree of hormone dependence or independence. Such an approach to classification of breast cancer would be a distinct

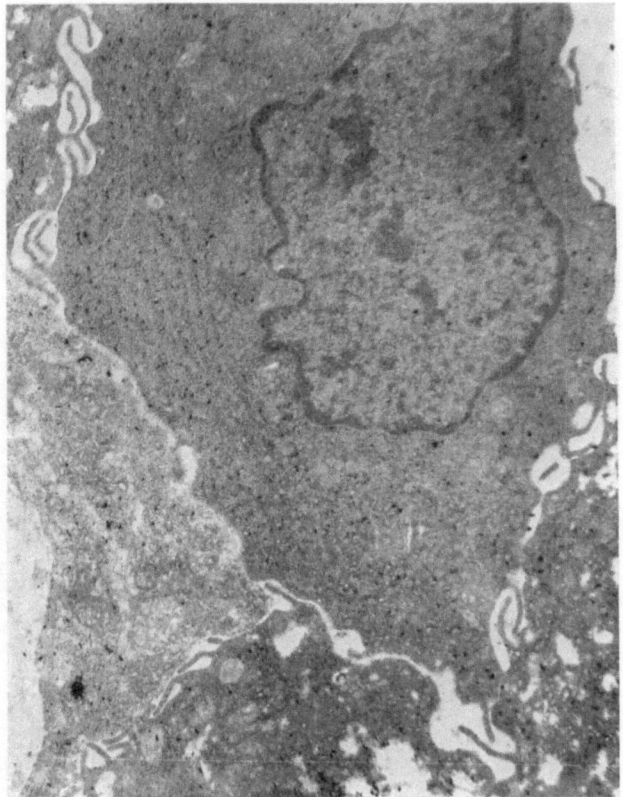

Fig. 5. Ductular carcinoma: Acid phosphatase activity localized diffusely throughout the cytoplasm. ($\times$10,600)

advantage over those in current vogue, all of which are a cumbersome combination of gross, histogenetic and histological characteristics, and biological behavior.

The foregoing brief review emphasizes the numerous approaches currently employed towards the understanding and prediction of the biological behavior of breast cancers. Although the major emphasis of pathologic studies continues to be morphologic, it is increasingly clear that morphologic methods alone do not possess the degree of accuracy necessary for optimal clinical management. While functional approaches to prognostication offer some promise, they too are limited when applied without the support of morphologic methods. The trend of modern clinicopathologic research in breast cancer is toward the combination of both morphologic and functional methodologies. Such studies will very probably lead to a sounder system for classification of breast cancers as well as a more rational approach to their therapy and management.

References

1. RICHTER, G. O., DOCKERTY, M. B., CLAGETT, O. T.: Diffuse infiltrating scirrhous carcinoma of the breast. Special consideration of the single-filing phenomenon. Cancer (Philad.) **20**, 363 (1967).
2. TAYLOR, H. B., NORRIS, H. J.: Well-differentiated carcinoma of the breast. Cancer (Philad.) **25**, 687 (1970).
3. CHRISTOPHERSON, W. M.: Prognosis of breast cancer based on pathologic type. Cancer (Philad.) **24**, 1179 (1969).
4. FOOTE, F. W., JR., STEWART, F. W.: A histologic classification of carcinoma of the breast. Surgery **19**, 74 (1946).
5. SCARFF, R. W., TORLONI, H.: Histological typing of breast tumors. International Histological Classification of Tumors 2, WHO Chron. (1968).
6. McDIVITT, R. W., STEWART, F. W., BERG, J. W.: Tumors of the Breast, 2nd series, fascicle 2. Washington D. C.: AFIP 1968.
7. HARTVEIT, F.: Prognostic typing in breast cancer. Brit. med. J. **4**, 253 (1971).
8. POTTER, J. F., SLIMBAUGH, W. P., WOODWARD, S. C.: Can breast carcinoma be anticipated? A follow-up of benign breast biopsies. Ann. Surg. **167**, 829 (1968).
9. HAYWARD, J. L.: The presymptomatic diagnosis of breast cancer. Proc. roy. Soc. Med. **59**, 1204 (1966).
10. BULBROOK, R. D., HAYWARD, J. L., THOMAS, B. S.: The relation between the urinary 17-hydroxycorticosteroids and 11-deoxy-17-oxosteroids and the fate of patients after mastectomy. Lancet **1964 I**, 945.
11. STANLEY, M. A., BIGHAM, D. A., COX, R. I., KIRKLAND, J. A., OPIT, L. J.: Sex-chromatin anomalies in female patients with breast carcinoma. Lancet **1966 I**, 690.
12. BLACK, M. M., KERPE, S., SPEER, F. D.: Lymph node structure in patients with cancer of the breast. Amer. J. Path. **29**, 505 (1953).
13. ANASTASSIADES, O. TH., PRYCE, D. M.: Immunological significance of the morphological changes in lymph nodes draining breast cancer. Brit. J. Cancer **20**, 239 (1966).
14. HAMLIN, I. M. E.: Possible host resistance in carcinoma of the breast: a histological study. Brit. J. Cancer **22**, 383 (1968).
15. BRIGHTMORE, T. G. J., GREENING, W. P., HAMLIN, I.: An analysis of clinical and histopathological features in 101 cases of carcinoma of breast in women under 35 years of age. Brit. J. Cancer **24**, 644 (1970).
16. BERG, J. W.: Inflammation and prognosis in breast cancer. Cancer (Philad.) **12**, 714 (1959).
17. KISTER, S. J., SOMMERS, S. C., HAAGENSEN, C. D., FRIEDELL, G. H., COOLEY, E., VARMA, A.: Nuclear grade and sinus histiocytosis in cancer of the breast. Cancer (Philad.) **23**, 570 (1969).
18. SOMMERS, S. C.: Histologic changes in incipient carcinoma of the breast. Cancer (Philad.) **23**, 822 (1969).
19. BLACK, M. M., SPEER, F. D.: Nuclear structure in cancer tissues. Surg. Gynec. Obstet. **105**, 97 (1957).
20. LEMON, H. M.: Endocrine influences on human mammary cancer formation. Cancer (Philad.) **23**, 781 (1969).
21. BRAUNSBERG, H., IRVINE, W. T., JAMES, V. H. T.: A comparison of steroid hormone concentrations in human tissues including breast cancer. Brit. J. Cancer **21**, 714 (1967).
22. QUINCEY, R. V., GRAY, C. H.: Uptake of [1,2-³H] 17α-methyltestosterone by breast carcinoma and other tissues of human subjects. Brit. J. Cancer **20**, 271 (1966).
23. FECHNER, R. E.: Breast cancer during oral contraceptive therapy. Cancer (Philad.) **26**, 1204 (1970).
24. GOLDENBERG, V. E., WIEGENSTEIN, L., MOTTET, N. K.: Florid breast fibroadenomas in patients taking hormonal oral contraceptives. Amer. J. clin. Path. **49**, 52 (1968).

25. Symmers, W. St. C.: Carcinoma of breast in trans-sexual individuals after surgical and hormonal interference with the primary and secondary sex characteristics. Brit. med. J. 2, 83 (1968).
26. Chalstrey, L. J., Benjamin, B.: High incidence of breast cancer in thyroid cancer patients. Brit. J. Cancer 20, 670 (1966).
27. Humphrey, L. J., Swerdlow, M.: The relationship of breast disease to thyroid disease. Cancer (Philad.) 17, 1170 (1964).
28. Murad, T. M., Greider, M. H., Scarpelli, D. G.: The ultrastructure of human mammary fibroadenoma. Amer. J. Path. 51, 663 (1967).
29. Murad, T. M.: A proposed histochemical and electron microscopic classification of human breast cancer according to cell of origin. Cancer (Philad.) 27, 288 (1971).
30. Murad, T. M.: Cytologic differentiation of carcinoma of the breast by electron microscopy. Acta cytol. (Philad.) 15, 400 (1971).
31. Hamperl, H.: The myothelia (myoepithelial cells) normal state, regressive changes; hyperplasia; tumors. In: Current Topics in Pathology 53, 162 (1970).
32. Pretlow, T. G., Boone, C. W.: Separation of mammalian cells using programmed gradient sedimentation. Exp. Mol. Path. 11, 139 (1969).
33. Pretlow, T. G., Pichichero, M. E., Hyams, L.: Separation of lymphocytes and macrophages from suspensions of guinea pig peritonitis exudate cells using programmed gradient sedimentation. Amer. J. Path. 63, 255 (1971).

Hormonal Dependency of Breast Cancer

E. V. Jensen, G. E. Block, S. Smith and E. R. DeSombre

Introduction

After the original demonstration of the striking remissions of breast cancer which follow removal of the ovaries of premenopausal women [1] or the adrenal glands of postmenopausal patients [2], it has become established that hormone deprivation affords effective, though often temporary, therapy for some but not all individuals with advanced breast cancer. Clinical experience has shown that about half the younger patients can expect benefit from ovariectomy, but a much smaller fraction (20—25%) of postmenopausal patients with breast cancer respond to adrenalectomy or hypophysectomy. A method of predicting *a priori* which breast cancers are of a hormone-dependent type would greatly enhance the usefulness of endocrine ablation, especially adrenalectomy in the older patient. One could restrict its application to those individuals in which it has a reasonable chance of success, thus sparing the majority of patients the trauma of major surgery which cannot help them and which renders them less able to tolerate alternative types of therapy. It now appears that the objective may be attained by determining the estrogen receptor content of a specimen of the tumor.

The two types of breast neoplasms, hormone-dependent and hormone-independent, have their counterparts in normal mammalian tissues, some of which require steroid hormones for their growth or function and some of which do not. An important characteristic of hormone-dependent or hormone-responsive tissues is their content of specific steroid-binding proteins, first recognized in the case of estrogens by the striking affinity of "target" tissues for tritiated estradiol or hexestrol, both *in vivo* and *in vitro*, and characterized most informatively by sedimentation of the estrogen-receptor complexes in sucrose density gradients. On the basis of contributions from many laboratories [3] it now appears that all classes of steroid hormones interact with their respective target tissues by similar two-step mechanisms, in which the hormone combines with an extranuclear receptor protein, inducing its translocation to the nucleus. Here the hormone-receptor complex accumulates in the chromatin and in some way initiates or accelerates biosynthetic processes, especially transcription. In the case of estrogens, migration to the nucleus is accompanied or probably preceded by conversion of the receptor protein to an active form, recognizable by a change in sedimentation properties.

The availability of detailed information about the interaction of estrogenic hormones with uterine tissue has provided a basis for comparing hormone-dependent with autonomous cancers. Soon after the original observations of the characteristic affinity of target tissues for estrogenic hormones, Folca, Glascock and Irvine [4] injected tritiated hexestrol into breast cancer patients, just prior to adrenalectomy, and observed that the uptake of radioactive hormone by the tumor, as compared to that of skeletal muscle, was greater in four patients who experienced remissions than in six patients who did not respond. Subsequent studies confirmed the ability of some human breast tumors to concentrate estrogenic hormones *in vivo* [5—8] and *in vitro* [9—11, 23, 24].

In contrast to their non-dependent counterparts, certain hormone-dependent rat mammary tumors were found to resemble rat uterus in their specific binding of estradiol, both *in vivo* and *in vitro* [12—18], and to contain a similar 8 S extranuclear receptor protein with a 4 S binding unit which serves as the precursor of the 5 S estradiol-receptor complex present in the nucleus [19, 20].

The foregoing indications of similarity in estrogen binding by hormone-dependent mammary tumors with that shown by estrogen target tissues suggested that the receptor content of human breast cancer specimens might provide an index for predicting which patients might benefit from ablative endocrine therapy. In 1966 we began such a study including both individuals with metastatic cancer, who were about to undergo endocrine therapy, and mastectomy patients in order to characterize for future reference the primary tumors of those patients in whom metastases might later appear.

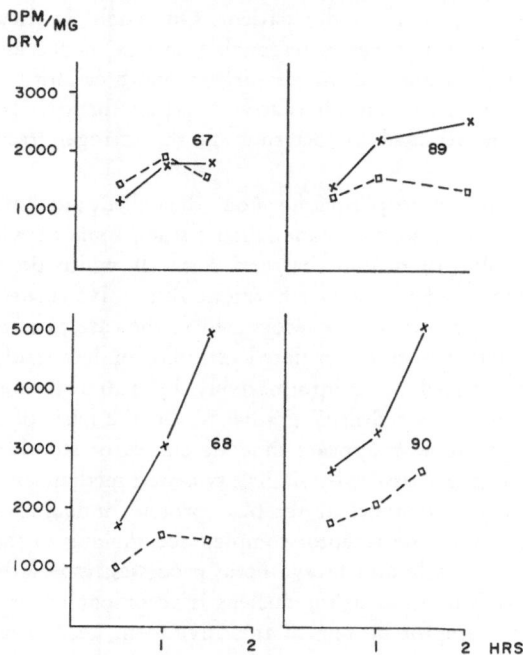

Fig. 1. One negative and three positive radioactivity uptake patterns for human breast cancer slices incubated at 37° C in 0.1 nM tritiated estradiol in the absence (solid line) or presence (broken line) of 10 µM Parke-Davis CI-628 in Krebs-Ringer-Henseleit glucose buffer, pH 7.3

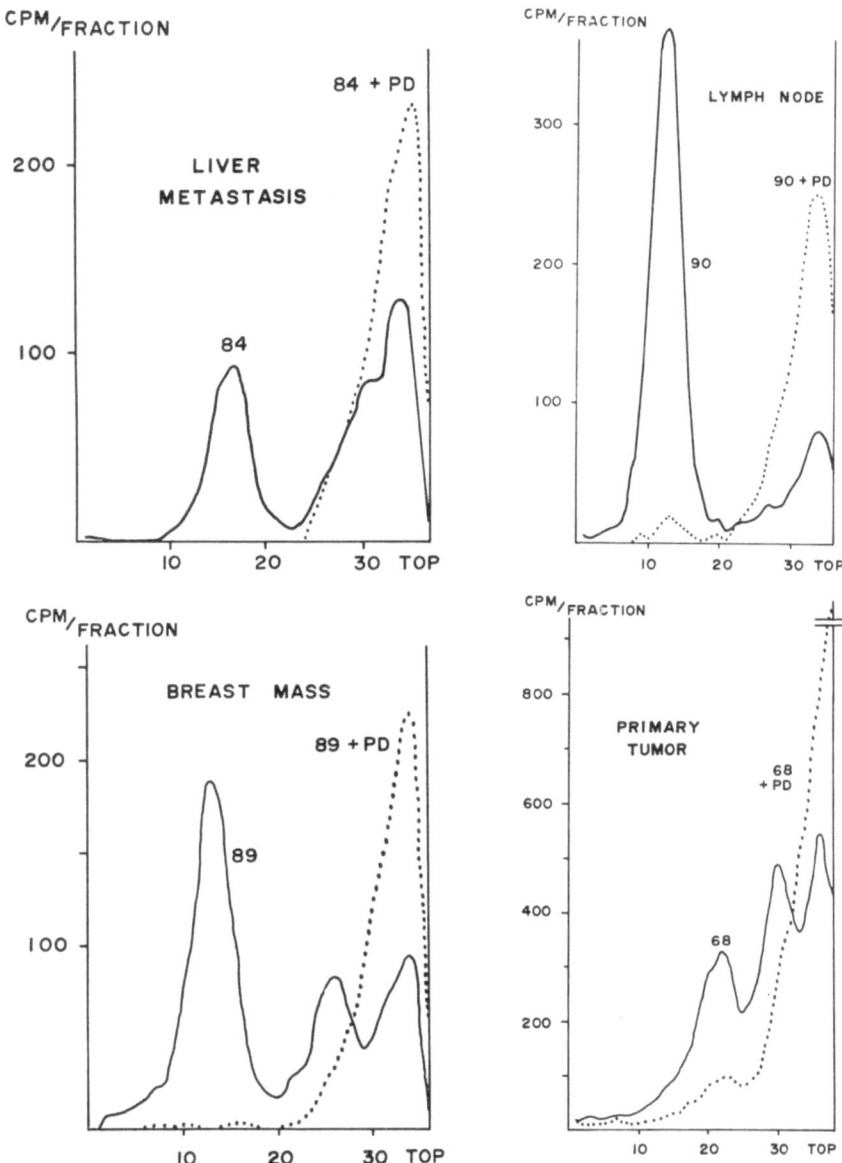

Fig. 2. Typical sedimentation patterns in sucrose gradients of positive human breast cancer cytosols containing 0.5 nM tritiated estradiol (2 nM for #68) in the absence (solid line) or presence (dotted line) of 0.2 μM PD CI-628. Some tumor cytosols show only 8 S complex in low salt gradients; others show varying amounts of 4 S sub-unit as well. Negative tumor cytosols show patterns similar to those illustrated for positive tumors plus PD CI-628, with no significant effect of the inhibitor

Estrogen Binding by Human Breast Cancers

In the earlier experiments, human breast cancer specimens were characterized by incubating 0.5 mm slices of the tumor tissue at 37° C in dilute (0.1 nM) solutions of tritiated estradiol in Krebs-Ringer-Henseleit buffer in the presence and absence of a specific binding inhibitor, either nafoxidine (Upjohn 11,100) or Parke-Davis CI-628 [21]. Typical negative (No. 67) and positive (Nos. 68, 89, 90) uptake patterns are illustrated in Fig. 1. Because of the variability in the number of cancer cells in different tumor specimens, the difference in estradiol incorporation in the presence or absence of the inhibitor is more significant than the actual magnitude of the uptake.

The uptake inhibition procedure provides a convenient means for characterizing breast cancers, but it is subject to two limitations. First, the tumor specimen must be sufficiently large (> 0.5 g) to provide at least five tissue slices for each time point, so

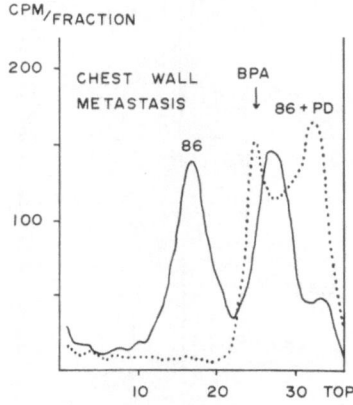

Fig. 3. Sedimentation pattern of a positive human breast cancer cytosol which contains serum protein. Because estradiol in excess of receptor capacity was not added, non-specific binding at 4.6 S is observed only when specific binding is eliminated by the inhibitor. BPA indicates the position of bovine plasma albumin marker

that variation due to heterogeneity of the cancer tissue can be minimized. Second, only fresh tumor specimens can be used; freezing renders the cells permeable to the extranuclear receptor protein which leaches out into the incubation medium and is not available for fixation of the hormone in the nucleus.

It was later found that direct estimation of the extranuclear receptor by sucrose gradient ultracentrifugation of the tumor cytosol after addition of excess tritiated estradiol provides a method of tumor characterization which is applicable to small (200 mg) samples of either fresh or frozen tissue. As illustrated in Fig. 2, the estradiol-receptor complex of some human breast cancer cytosols sediments in a low salt sucrose gradient entirely in an 8 S form (Nos. 84, 90) while with other cancers the complex exists partly in a 4 S form (Nos. 68, 89). This may represent the 4 S subunit of the 8 S receptor which in adult but not immature rat uterus has been found to remain partially in the 4 S form in low salt gradients [22]. Both of these specific sedimentation peaks can be distinguished from weak non-specific (4.6 S) binding to serum proteins, which is seen with some cancer specimens (Fig. 3), by their sensitivity to the specific binding inhibitor, Parke Davis CI-628. With negative tumor specimens, identical sedimentation patterns are observed in the presence or absence of the inhibitor, with the radioactive estradiol appearing either at the top of the tube as illustrated, or, if serum proteins are present, partly bound in the 4.6 S region.

The more recent cancer specimens were all evaluated by the sedimentation procedure; in those cases where sufficient sample was available, slice uptake also was carried out with excellent agreement between the two methods. More complete description of experimental detail is given elsewhere [21].

Results and Clinical Correlations

As summarized in Table 1, the 117 primary tumors studied were about equally divided between those which contained receptor and those which did not, with a small number of borderline cases. With 57 metastatic tumors, about twice as many negative as positive patterns were observed. In most cases where more than one tumor specimen (primary and metastasis or two or more metastases) was obtained from the same patient, all samples showed similar patterns, but in one instance clear evidence of both positive and negative metastases in the same patient was observed.

Table 1. Occurrence of estrogen receptors in human breast cancers [a]

	Positive	Borderline	Negative	Both positive and negative
Primary tumors	56	8	53	
Without metastases	45	5	42	
With metastases [b]	11	3	11	
Metastatic tumors	18	4	34	1 [c]

[a] Presence of receptor determined by estradiol uptake in tumor slices and/or sedimentation peak on sucrose gradient centrifugation of cytosol.

[b] Seventeen of the patients whose primary tumors were accompanied by metastases received endocrine therapy and are included in Table 2. Two other mastectomy patients developed subsequent metastases.

[c] In one case, where four different metastatic specimens were examined, two axillary lymph nodes were positive and two distant metastases were negative. Because this patient also had cardiac disease, from which she died, no ablative endocrine therapy was carried out.

Because of the higher incidence of remission after ovariectomy in premenopausal breast cancer patients than after adrenalectomy in older patients, one might expect that receptor-containing tumors would be more prevalent in the younger age group. On the basis of the patients studied so far, this does not seem to be the case. The median age for the 56 patients with positive primary tumors was 63 (range 34—83), as compared to a median age of 56 (range 32—86) for the 53 negative patients. The median age of the 18 patients with positive metastatic tumors was 52 (range 32—69) and that for the 34 patients with negative metastases was 51 (range 25—71).

Of the 81 patients with metastatic disease studied, 54 received some type of endocrine therapy under conditions permitting evaluation of clinical response. In most instances treatment commenced at the time the tumor was characterized, but in a few

Table 2. Correlation of receptor presence with clinical response [a]

Receptor test:		Positive		Borderline		Negative	
Therapy [b]	Specimen examined	R	F	R	F	R	F
Adrenalectomy [c]	Primary	4		2		4	
	Metastasis	4	3 [d]	1		1	12
Hypophysectomy	Primary					2	
	Metastasis	1				4	
Oophorectomy [e]	Primary	1		1		1	
	Metastasis				1	5	
Androgen	Primary					1	
	Metastasis	1					
Estrogen plus progestin	Primary	1	1				
Parke-Davis CI-628	Metastasis	1				1	
Diethylstilbestrol	Primary					1	
Total		13	4	1	4	1	31

[a] R = objective remission, F = failure to respond.

[b] With one positive, one borderline and three negative adrenalectomy patients, as well as one negative hypophysectomy, one negative androgen and one negative diethylstilbestrol therapy, treatment was carried out 4 to 12 months after the tumor specimen was examined. With one borderline adrenalectomy, one negative hypophysectomy and three negative oophorectomy-plus androgen patients, the tumor specimen was examined 4 to 12 months after unsuccessful therapy was instituted.

[c] Six positive, two borderline and six negative adrenalectomy patients had accompanying oophorectomy or, in two cases, radiation castration.

[d] One of these "false positive" patients had experienced remission after oophorectomy 6 months earlier and showed subjective but not objective remission to adrenalectomy. Another had shown remission to oophorectomy 19 months earlier.

[e] One positive and four negative oophorectomy patients also received androgen following oophorectomy.

cases it was carried out either before or after the tumor sample was taken for study. As summarized in Table 2, of 32 patients whose cancers showed negative patterns, only one experienced remission after endocrine therapy (adrenalectomy). In contrast, 13 out of 17 patients whose cancers showed evidence of receptor content experienced objective remission. The failure of some patients with positive patterns is understandable if one considers that it is possible, although apparently not common, to have a mixed population of positive and negative metastases. In such cases, the pattern observed may be either positive or negative, depending on which metastasis is obtained for study, but the endocrine treatment will be a failure because the negative metastases will be unresponsive.

Summary

On the basis of the foregoing studies, summarized in Table 3, it would appear that human breast cancers fall into two categories, those which contain significant amounts of the estrogen receptor protein and those which do not. These can be distinguished by examination of a cancer specimen *in vitro*. A few borderline cases are found. In case of metastatic disease, most but not all patients with receptor-containing tumors may expect benefit from endocrine therapy. But if a cancer shows no distinct evidence of estrogen receptors, that patient has little chance of remission and probably can be spared the trauma of adrenalectomy or other ablative therapy.

Table 3. Summary of objective remissions

	Ablation-47	Hormone-7	Overall-54
Positive	10/13	3/4	13/17
Borderline	1/ 5		1/ 5
Negative	1/29	0/3	1/32

Acknowledgement

The earlier investigations of estrogen receptors in mammary tumors were supported by research grant P-422 from the American Cancer Society and the later studies by USPHS contract PH 43-66-945 from the National Cancer Institute.

References

1. BEATSON, G. T.: On the treatment of inoperable cases of carcinoma of the mamma: Suggestions for a new method of treatment with illustrative cases. Lancet 1896 II, 104.
2. HUGGINS, C., BERGENSTAL, D. M.: Inhibition of human mammary and prostatic cancer by adrenalectomy. Cancer Res. 12, 134 (1952).
3. JENSEN, E. V., DE SOMBRE, E. R.: Mechanism of action of the female sex hormones. Ann. Rev. Biochem. 41, 203 (1972).
4. FOLCA, P. J., GLASCOCK, R. F., IRVINE, W. T.: Studies with tritium-labeled hexoestrol in advanced breast cancer. Lancet 1961 II, 796.
5. DEMETRIOU, J. A., CROWLEY, L. G., KUCHINSKY, S., DONOVAN, A. J., KOTIN, P., MACDONALD, I.: Radioactive estrogens in tissues of postmenopausal women with breast neoplasms. Cancer Res. 24, 926 (1964).
6. PEARLMAN, W. H., DE HERTOGH, R., LAUMAS, K. R., BRUEGGMANN, J. A., PEARLMAN, M. R. J.: Metabolism and tissue uptake of steroid sex hormones in patients with advanced carcinoma of the breast and in normal rats. In: Steroid Dynamics. Eds.: PINCUS, G., NAKAO, T., and TAIT, J. F.: New York: Academic Press 1966, p. 159.
7. BRAUNSBERG, H., IRVINE, W. T., JAMES, V. H. T.: A comparison of steroid hormone concentrations in human tissues including breast cancer. Brit. J. Cancer 21, 714 (1967).
8. DESHPANDE, N., JENSEN, V., BULBROOK, R. D., BERNE, T., ELLIS, F.: Accumulation of tritiated oestradiol by human breast tissue. Steroids 10, 219 (1967).
9. SANDER, S.: The in vitro uptake of oestradiol in biopsies from 25 breast cancer patients. Acta path. microbiol. scand. 74, 301 (1968).
10. JOHANSSON, H., TERENIUS, L., THORÉN, L.: The binding of estradiol-17β to human breast cancers and other tissues in vitro. Cancer Res. 30, 692 (1970).
11. KORENMAN, S. G., DUKES, B. A.: Specific estrogen binding by the cytoplasm of human breast carcinoma. J. clin. Endocr. 30, 639 (1970).
12. KING, R. J. B., COWAN, D. M., INMAN, D. R.: The uptake of [6,7-^{3}H] oestradiol by dimethylbenzanthracene-induced rat mammary tumours. J. Endocr. 32, 83 (1965).
13. JENSEN, E. V.: The mechanism of estrogen action in relation to carcinogenesis. Proc. Canad. Cancer Res. Conf. 6, 143 (1965).
14. MOBBS, B. G.: The uptake of tritiated oestradiol by dimethylbenzanthracene-induced mammary tumours of the rat. J. Endocr. 36, 409 (1966).

15. Mobbs, B. G.: The uptake of simultaneously adminstered [³H] oestradiol and [¹⁴C] progesterone by dimethylbenzanthracene-induced rat mammary tumours. J. Endocr. **41**, 339 (1968).

16. Jensen, E. V., De Sombre, E. R., Jungblut, P. W.: Estrogen receptors in hormone-responsive tissues and tumors. In: Endogenous Factors Influencing Host-Tumor Balance. Eds.: Wissler, R. W., Dao, T. L., and Wood, S., Jr., p. 15, p. 68. Chicago: University of Chicago Press 1967.

17. Sander, S., Attramadal, A.: The *in vivo* uptake of oestradiol-17β by hormone responsive and unresponsive breast tumours of the rat. Acta path. microbiol. scand. **74**, 169 (1968).

18. Sander, S.: The *in vitro* uptake of oestradiol in DMBA-induced breast tumours of the rat. Acta path. microbiol. scand. **75**, 520 (1969).

19. Kyser, K. A.: The tissue, subcellular and molecular binding of estradiol to dimethylbenzathracene-induced rat mammary tumor. University of Chicago: Ph.D. Dissertation 1970.

20. McGuire, W. L., Julian, J. A.: Comparison of macromolecular binding of estradiol in hormone-dependent and hormone-independent rat mammary carcinoma. Cancer Res. **31**, 1440 (1971).

21. Jensen, E. V., Block, G. E., Smith, S., Kyser, K., De Sombre, E. R.: Estrogen receptors and breast cancer response to adrenalectomy. In: Prediction of Response in Cancer Therapy, National Cancer Institute Monograph No. 34. Ed.: Hall, T. C. Washington, D. C.: U. S. Government Printing Office 1971, p. 55.

22. Steggles, A. W., King, R. J. B.: The use of protamine to study [6,7-³H] oestradiol-17β binding in rat uterus. Biochem. J. **118**, 695 (1970).

23. Hähnel, R., Twaddle, E., Vivian, A. B.: Estrogen receptors in human breast cancer 2. *In vitro* binding of estradiol by benign and malignant tumors. Steroids **18**, 681 (1971).

24. James, F., James, V. H. T., Carter, A. E., Irvine, W. T.: A comparison of *in vivo* and *in vitro* uptake of estradiol by human breast tumors and the relationship to steroid excretion. Cancer Res. **31**, 1268 (1971).

Is there Evidence that Immunity Influences Tumor-Host Balance in Breast Cancer?

G. H. Heppner

That immune responses to breast cancer in humans might be involved in regulation of tumor growth was first suspected on the basis of histological observations. Berg described a characteristic plasma cell-lymphocytic infiltration occurring in 73% of anaplastic infiltrating duct carcinomas which responded well to treatment [1]. This type of infiltrate, which was associated with degenerating changes in the cancer cells, was found in only 27% of cases selected at random and in 30% of similar cancers with fatal outcome. Lymphocytic infiltrations were also noted to be more frequent in tumors from patients living at least 10 years after surgical removal than in patients who were not cured by surgery [2]. Direct evidence that immune responses can influence the balance between breast cancer and tumor host is lacking; however, studies on mammary tumors of mice, and more recently of humans, strongly suggest that this is so. This paper is a brief review of the basic features of mouse mammary tumor immunology, including the types of antigens found, the influence of mammary tumor virus (MTV) infection on the capacity to respond to these antigens, and the types of anti-tumor immune responses detected by *in vitro* techniques. In addition, the correlation between the growth of mammary tumors and the detection of immune responses will be discussed. Finally recent studies on immune responses to breast cancer in humans will be described.

Transplantation Immunity to Mouse Mammary Tumors

Most of the work on the immunogenicity of mouse mammary cancer has been done with tumors arising in mice infected with MTV. Although early attempts to show tumor-associated antigenicity of these tumors were not successful [3, 4], more recent work has substantiated the phenomenon [5—7]. It has become apparent, however, that infection with MTV plays an important role in induction of transplantation immunity to mammary tumor antigens. Mice which are free of the virus can be easily immunized to cells of a syngeneic, MTV-induced tumor. MTV-infected mice, which receive virus shortly after birth in their mother's milk, are much more difficult to immunize, and in general, show a greater tendency than do MTV-free mice to support growth of transplanted mammary tumor cells [5—9]. In addition, the pattern of immune reactivity to tumor cells differs with the status of MTV infection. Immunity which is induced in virus-free mice extends to all syngeneic mammary tumors, that is, it is cross-reacting, whereas infected mice are generally able to show resistance only to the tumor used for immunization [5, 7, 10]. Indeed, multiple tumors initially arising in the same animal may not cross-react in virus infected mice [11].

On the basis of the differences between MTV-infected and free mice in immune reactivity to mammary tumors, WEISS and MORTON [5, 9] independently proposed that neonatal infection with that virus induced a state of tolerance to MTV and associated antigens. Thus, only virus free mice could recognize those antigens, which, in analogy to the findings with other virus-induced tumors, were common to all mammary tumors and hence induced cross-reacting immunity. The fact that infected mice could be immunized, in a non-cross-reacting pattern, to mammary tumors showed that these tumors had additional tumor antigens, which, in analogy to chemically-induced tumors, were unique to each tumor [12, 13].

In Vitro Detection of Immune Responses to Mouse Mammary Tumors

All the above conclusions on the immunogenicity of mouse mammary tumors are derived from *in vivo* studies using growth of transplanted, or autochthonous, tumors as an endpoint for immune resistance. It is obvious that such an approach is not possible for study of human breast cancer. In addition, the various types of immune responses involved in the total reaction to a tumor can be independently analyzed only with difficulty in *in vivo* experiments. For these reasons we have been studying immune responses to breast cancer *in vitro,* using colony inhibition and cytotoxicity techniques originally described by the HELLSTRÖMS [14—16]. These tests measure the ability of immune factors to influence the viability and/or multiplication of tumor cells under tissue culture conditions.

As with other solid tumors, immune resistance to mammary tumors seems to be cell-mediated and can be passively transferred from immunized to non-sensitized animals with lymph node or peritoneal washing cells [17]. Evidence for this cell-mediated immunity was also obtained from *in vitro* experiments showing that lymph node cells from either autochthonous hosts, or from mice immunized by implantation and subsequent removal of living tumor cells, could inhibit growth of mammary tumor cells [15, 18]. The pattern of immune reactivity was very similar to what had earlier been described *in vivo:* lymph node cells from mice infected neonatally with MTV could only react against cells of the immunizing tumor, whereas lymph node cells from MTV-free mice were capable of cross-reacting. A summary of our data on detection of cell-mediated immunity *in vitro* is presented in Table 1.

In addition to cell-mediated immunity, humoral, cytotoxic immune responses to mammary tumor antigens have been detected [19]. However, ATTIA and WEISS [20] reported that increased susceptibility, capable of being passively transferred by serum, was sometimes seen in mice "immunized" to mammary tumors. This is similar to the phenomenon of immune enhancement described for allogeneic systems [21]. One of the hypotheses to explain enhancement involves efferent blocking of cell-mediated immunity by serum antibody [22]. Accordingly, serum from either autochthonous or sensitized mice was frequently found capable of neutralizing the ability of immune lymph node cells to inhibit growth of mammary tumor cells [23]. This blocking effect was specific for mammary tumors, and in the case of MTV-infected donors, for the immunizing tumor. More detailed analysis in other systems suggests

Table 1. Summary of colony inhibition and microcytotoxicity experiments with breast tumors: cell-mediated immunity

Source of lymphocytes	Source of tumor	Proportion of experiments in which significant cellular immunity detected
MTV-infected mice	Immunizing tumor	46/54 (85.2%)
	Another mouse mammary tumor	1/30 (3.3%)
MTV-free mice	Immunizing tumor	29/32 (90.6%)
	Another mouse mammary tumor	13/23 (56.5%)
Human breast cancer patient	Own tumor	6/9 (66.7%)
	Another human breast carcinoma	9/12 (75.0%)

Table 2. Summary of colony inhibition and microcytotoxicity experiments with breast tumors: blocking antibody

Source of serum	Source of tumor	Proportion of experiments in which significant blocking of cellular immunity detected
MTV-infected mice	Immunizing tumor	25/38 (65.9%)
	Another mouse mammary tumor	1/14 (7.1%)
MTV-free mice	Immunizing tumor	9/15 (60.0%)
	Another mouse mammary tumor	not enough tests
Human breast cancer patient	Own tumor	5/7 (71.4%)
	Another human breast carcinoma	3/6 (50.0%)

that the blocking factor is an antibody, or possibly, an antigen-antibody complex [24]. Table 2 summarizes our *in vitro* experiments designed to detect blocking factor in mammary tumor systems.

More recently another factor has been found in sera from mice immunized to mammary tumors. This factor, which is detectable with about one-fourth of the tumors, is capable of rendering lymph node cells from non-sensitized mice cytotoxic for mammary tumor cells in colony inhibition experiments [25]. It is not by itself cytotoxic. No information is yet available on the nature of this factor.

Correlation between Immune Responses Detected *in Vitro* and Growth of Mouse Mammary Tumors *in Vivo*

In vitro experiments show that a variety of immune responses can be detected in mice against autochthonous or syngeneic mammary tumors. The next step is to see whether these responses can affect growth of tumors *in vivo*. That this is probably so is shown by the transplantation experiments discussed earlier and by studies demonstrating that either specific or non-specific immunotherapy can retard development or growth of even autochthonous tumors [7, 19, 26—28]. However, the complexity of immune responses detected *in vitro* suggests that the total immune regulation of tumor growth is made up of a "balance" of responses, with the direction of effect dependent upon the relative concentrations of cytotoxic and blocking factors. So far we have examined this proposition only for cell-mediated cytotoxicity and blocking antibody.

To study the roles of cellular immunity and blocking antibody in regulating growth of mammary tumors, it would be helpful to have a means of independently regulating the development of these two immune responses. A partial approach to this problem was provided by the observation of CALABRESI [29] that early administration, in relatively low doses, of cytosine arabinoside (are-C) would inhibit antibody production in mice without suppressing cellular immunity. We therefore injected C3H/HeJ (MTV-infected) mice with cells of a syngeneic mammary tumor and then treated with ara-C for a total of 5 days. Tumors in animals receiving relatively low doses of ara-C grew out about 2 weeks later than in controls, whereas tumors in mice receiving high doses of drug appeared about 2 weeks earlier. Parallel *in vitro* experiments showed that anti-tumor, cell-mediated immunity, which in control mice was detected for 1—2 weeks after tumor cell injection before falling to undetectable levels, was found for 3—4 weeks in mice given low doses of drug. Cell-mediated immunity was completely suppressed by high doses of drug. Blocking immunity, which was detected at all times tested in control mice, was suppressed for 2 weeks in the mice given low doses of ara-C and completely suppressed in mice given high doses [30].

Thus, suppression of cellular (and blocking) immunity was associated with rapid tumor growth. Suppression of blocking immunity only was associated with retarded tumor growth.

Further evidence that the effects of ara-C on growth of syngeneic mammary tumor cells were related to suppression of immune reactivity was provided by experiments on a tumor outgrowth line which was non-immunogenic, in that it was unable to induce cellular immunity in virus infected mice, as detected by *in vitro* colony inhibition tests. Ara-C treatment of mice given cells from this outgrowth had no effect on tumor growth, regardless of whether high or low doses of drug were used.

The experiments with ara-C, therefore, tend to support the hypothesis that part of the regulation of mammary tumor growth in mice is based on a balance between cell-mediated and blocking immunity.

Another approach to the problem of determining the effects on tumor growth of cellular versus blocking immunity comes from observations on surgery and tumor immunity. It has long been appreciated that maximal transplantation resistance to tumor cells is seen in animals 1 week or more after surgical removal of an immunizing, live implant of tumor cells [31, 32]. We therefore injected mice with measured suspensions of viable, syngeneic tumor cells. The tumors were allowed to grow out to a size of 10 mm² in surface area. Cellular and blocking immune reactions were measured *in vitro* with colony inhibition tests after either complete surgical removal of these tumors, sham surgical removal, or no surgery.

Cell-mediated immunity was detected 10—15 days after surgery in 12 of 13 experiments in the complete removal group, 12 of 15 experiments in the sham removal group, but in only 7 of 17 experiments in mice which had no surgery and still bore their tumors [33].

Blocking antibody was measured at 2 times—1—5 days and 10—15 days—after surgery. It was detected with equal frequency in all 3 groups of mice when measured at the earlier times, but had fallen to significantly lower levels in the complete removal group, as compared to the other 2 groups, by 10—15 days after surgery [33].

Thus, heightened cellular immunity and diminishing blocking antibody were associated with increased transplantation resistance to tumor isografts. Interestingly, sham surgery had a stimulatory effect on cell-mediated immunity, although blocking antibody was not affected.

Finally, evidence that blocking immunity may play a role *in vivo* comes from studies on the effect of neonatal thymectomy on tumor development and tumor growth. MARTINEZ [34] was the first to show that removal of the thymus shortly after birth resulted in a suppression of the spontaneous development of mammary tumors in MTV-infected, adult female mice. This finding has been repeated a number of times, with some differences in the extent of tumor suppression, depending upon the strain of mice [35—39]. Although the correct explanation for this occurrence will probably be complex, comprising, in addition to immunological effects, developmental, hormonal, and nutritional factors, we have found that neonatally thymectomized mice are unable to make blocking antibody to syngeneic transplants of mammary tumors ([39] and unpublished observations). The cell-mediated response is as vigorous *in vitro* as is that of normal mice, although the total number of lymphocytes is reduced *in vivo*. Mammary tumor transplants also grow more slowly in the thymectomized mice than in controls [39]. Thus, once again *in vivo* tumor growth is correlated with *in vitro* measurement of tumor immune responses.

Detection of Immune Responses to Human Breast Cancer

Evidence that immune responses to tumor antigens in human breast carcinoma, as well as in other human tumors, may be similar to those detected in mice is only now being accumulated. Cell-mediated responses to autochthonous breast cancer have been detected by colony inhibition and microcytotoxicity tests [40], by inhibition of leucocyte migration with extracts of tumor cells [41], and by an interesting skin window technique in which the type of inflammatory exudate forming on a slide mounted with a cryostat section of autochthonous breast tumor is assessed [42]. The frequency of detection of cell-mediated reactivity to autochthonous tumors has varied with the technique used. Using colony inhibition and microcytotoxicity tests, the HELLSTRÖMS and co-workers have found immunity in 7 of 8 breast cancer patients [40]. Our own data with these tests give results of 6 of 9. These frequencies are similar to those found in mice when tested against their own tumors (Table 1).

In addition to cellular reactivity against autochthonous tumors, peripheral lymphocytes from breast cancer patients have been regularly found to inhibit growth of tumor cells from other breast tumors. The HELLSTRÖM group has found cross-reacting inhibition in 13 of 15 experiments [40], whereas we have done so in 9 of 12 tests. It has been suggested that breast cancer in humans may be associated with the presence of a milk-borne virus, similar to that of mouse mammary cancer [43]. The finding of cross-reactivity between human tumors does not support this hypothesis, since one would except that a woman who developed breast cancer would have a reactivity similar to that of a MTV-infected mouse. Alternatively, it may be that tolerance to virus associated antigens is less easily induced, or more easily broken, in humans than in mice. However, there is an important methodological difference in experiments between humans and mice, namely the lack of inbred humans. All tests for cross-reacting breast tumor immunity in humans have been done with allogeneic tumors. It is possible that some of the detected cross-reactivity could be a result of antigenic differences unrelated to tumor antigens.

Blocking factors capable of inhibiting cellular immunity to breast tumor antigens have also been found in sera from breast cancer patients. In a recent publication the HELLSTRÖMS et al. list a frequency of detection of 3 out of 5 in autochthonous tests and 10 of 17 in allogeneic experiments [44]. Our own data are 5 of 7 and 3 of 6, respectively (Table 2). Again the high degree of cross-reactivity in human experiments contrasts with the results of mouse experiments.

The HELLSTRÖMS and associates have also described another factor, which they call "unblocking" antibody, in the serum of 5 breast cancer patients who have had no recurrent disease at times ranging from $3^1/_2$ months to 4 years after treatment by surgery [45]. Sera from patients with metastatic breast carcinoma, when mixed with sera from these 5 patients, had no effect on cell-mediated destruction of breast cancer cells, whereas sera from patients with metastatic disease mixed with normal sera resulted in blocking of that immunity.

Immune Responses and the Tumor-Host Balance in Human Breast Cancer

Data on the correlation of immune responses, as measured by various procedures, and cancer growth is much more difficult to collect in humans than in mice. Ultimately, long term studies with close clinical observation and sequential determination of immune reactivity will be necessary. Modes of therapy will have to be considered. At this time it is only possible to state that the data so far reported on immunity versus tumor growth are promising. BLACK and LEIS [42] have recently demonstrated that inflammatory exudates characteristic of delayed hypersensitivity responses are more often induced to frozen autochthonous tumor cells in patients with Stage I breast carcinoma than in those with Stage II disease. This type of exudate was also positively correlated with lymphoreticuloendothelial reactions in both primary tumors and axillary lymph nodes. In vitro studies, however, indicate that cell-mediated immunity to tumor antigens by itself does not correlate well with extent of disease. Thus, the HELLSTRÖMS et al. find that lymphocyte-mediated destruction of either autochthonous or allogeneic breast tumor cells can almost always be detected, whether the donor of the lymphocytes has an actively growing tumor (7 of 8 experiments) or has been free of disease for some time (13 of 15 experiments) [40]. On the other hand, blocking antibody is most often detected in serum from tumor-bearing patients (9 of 12 experiments), and is absent in serum from patients free of clinical signs of disease (0 of 3 experiments) [44]. Our own data are extremely preliminary. So far, however, we have also found that cellular immunity is nearly always present regardless of the extent of disease. The exceptions to this rule are patients whose tumors have been surgically removed one week or less before the test (Table 3). Only

4 of 8 such patients showed detectable immunity. Patients who have either had no surgery, or whose surgery was greater than 1 week before the test, showed positive cellular reactions in 10 of 10 tests. Blocking immunity was detected in all patients within the first week of surgery. We unfortunately have not tested enough breast cancer patients with only local disease at greater than 1 week after surgery to attempt to correlate extent of disease with blocking immunity. In melanoma patients, how-

Table 3. Cellular and blocking immune responses to breast carcinoma in human patients

Time of surgery	Extent of disease	No. of patients positive/no. tested for:	
		Cellular immunity	Blocking antibody
Within 1 week	Local	1/3	3/3
	Regional or widespread	3/5	2/2
	Total	4/8	5/5
Beyond 1 week, or no surgery	Local	2/2	0/1
	Regional or widespread	8/8	5/6
	Total	10/10	5/7

ever, we have found that blocking antibody is not present in patients with local disease, but can be found in those with regional or widespread cancer (unpublished observations).

As mentioned previously, another factor, called "unblocking antibody" has been found in the sera of breast cancer patients who have remained symptomatically free of disease from $3^{1}/_{2}$ months to 4 years after surgery [45]. This factor also may be an indicator of clinical status.

Summary

Although the question of the role of immune responses in regulation of growth of breast cancer in humans is not yet resolved, there are signs that such responses are important. Cellular and humoral responses, similar to those detected in experimental mouse mammary tumors, can be demonstrated in breast cancer patients. Since some, at least, of these immune responses can be shown to be correlated with tumor growth in mice, it is likely that the same correlations will be found in humans. Preliminary data in humans are encouraging in this respect. The therapeutic potentialities of immune responses in breast cancer, however, remain to be determined.

Acknowledgements

I would like to especially thank Drs. KARL-ERIC and INGEGERD HELLSTRÖM, University of Washington Medical School, Seattle, Washington, and Dr. PAUL CALABRESI, Roger Williams General Hospital and Brown University, Providence, Rhode Island, in whose laboratories many of the experiments described in this paper were done. I would also like to thank Dr. LEO L. STOLBACH, Pondville Hospital, Waltham, Mass., Dr. FRANK CUMMINGS, Roger Williams General Hospital, Providence, R. I.,

Dr. MICHAEL BYRNE, Tufts University School of Medicine, Boston, Mass., and Dr. EUGENE McDONOUGH, Harvard Medical School, Boston, Mass. for their collaboration in experiments with human breast cancer. My thanks also go to Mrs. JANICE KOPP, Miss ELIZABETH SWANSON, Mrs. SHERRIE WILKE, and Miss GAIL STEVENS for skilled technical assistance. Some of the work reported here was done while I was a DAMON RUNYON post-doctoral fellow. This work was also supported by American Cancer Society institutional cancer grants to the University of Washington and to Brown University and by Grant GM 16538, United States Public Health Service (General Medical Sciences).

References

1. BERG, J. W.: Inflammation and prognosis in breast cancer. A search for host resistance. Cancer (Philad.) 12, 714 (1959).
2. LANE, M., GOKSEL, H., SALERNO, R. A., HAAGENSEN, C. D.: Clinico-pathologic analysis of the surgical curability of breast cancers: a minimum ten-year study of a personal series. Ann. Surg. 153, 483 (1961).
3. FOLEY, E. J.: Attempts to induce immunity against mammary adenocarcinoma in inbred mice. Cancer Res. 13, 835 (1953).
4. REVESZ, L.: Detection of antigenic differences in isologous host tumor systems by pretreatment with irradiated tumor cells. Cancer Res. 20, 443 (1960).
5. WEISS, D. W., LAVRIN, D. H., DEZFULIAN, M., VAAGE, J., BLAIR, P. B.: Studies on the immunology of spontaneous mammary carcinomas of mice. In: Viruses Inducing Cancer. Ed.: BURDETTE, W. J. Salt Lake City: University of Utah Press 1966, p. 138.
6. RIGGINS, R. S., PILCH, Y. J.: Immunity to spontaneous and methylcholanthrene-induced tumors in inbred mice. Cancer Res. 24, 1994 (1964).
7. VAAGE, J.: Immunologic and immunotherapeutic studies on spontaneous and transplanted mouse mammary carcinomas. In: Immunity and Tolerance in Oncogenesis. Ed.: SEVERI, L. Perugia (Italy): University of Perugia 1970, p. 1085.
8. BARRETT, M. K., DUNN, T. B.: Influence of the mammary tumor agent on the longevity of hosts bearing a transplanted tumor. J. nat. Cancer Inst. 13, 109 (1952).
9. MORTON, D. L.: Acquired immunological tolerance and carcinogenesis by the mammary tumor virus. I. Influence of neonatal infection with the mammary tumor virus on the growth of spontaneous mammary adenocarcinomas. J. nat. Cancer Inst. 42, 311 (1969).
10. WEISS, D. W., SHEN, A.: Immunology of spontaneous mammary tumors in mice. Cross-reacting immunogenicity of C3H tumors in C3Hf and C3H/2 mice. Proc. Amer. Ass. Cancer Res. 7, 75 (1966).
11. VAAGE, J., KALINOVSKY, T., OLSON, R.: Antigenic differences among virus-induced mouse mammary tumors arising spontaneously in the same C3H/Crgl host. Cancer Res. 29, 1452 (1969).
12. MORTON, D. L., MILLER, G. F., WOOD, D. A.: Demonstration of tumor-specific immunity against antigens unrelated to the mammary tumor virus in spontaneous mammary adenocarcinomas. J. nat. Cancer Inst. 42, 289 (1969).
13. VAAGE, J.: Nonvirus-associated antigens in virus-induced mouse mammary tumors. Cancer Res. 28, 2477 (1968).
14. HELLSTRÖM, I.: A colony inhibition (CI) technique for demonstration of tumor cell destruction by lymphoid cells in vitro. Int. J. Cancer 2, 65 (1967).
15. HEPPNER, G. H., KOPP, J. S.: A dilute agar colony inhibition (CI) test for studying cell-mediated immune responses against tumor cells. Int. J. Cancer 7, 26 (1971).
16. HELLSTRÖM, I., HELLSTRÖM, K. E.: Colony inhibition and cytotoxicity assays. In: In vitro Methods in Cell-Mediated Immunity. Eds.: BLOOM, B. R., and GLADE, P. R. New York: Academic Press 1971, p. 413.
17. ATTIA, A. M., DEOME, K. B., WEISS, D. W.: Immunology of spontaneous mammary carcinomas in mice. II. Resistance to rapidly and slowly developing tumors. Cancer Res. 25, 451 (1965).

18. HEPPNER, G. H., PIERCE, G.: In vitro demonstration of tumor-specific antigens in spontaneous mammary tumors of mice. Int. J. Cancer 4, 212 (1969).
19. IRIE, K., IRIE, R. F.: Immunological suppression of the occurrence of spontaneous mammary tumors in C3H/He mice. Nature (Lond.) 233, 133 (1971).
20. ATTIA, M. A. M., WEISS, D. W.: Immunology of spontaneous mammary carcinomas in mice. V. Acquired tumor resistance and enhancement in strain A mice infected with mammary tumor virus. Cancer Res. 26, 1787 (1966).
21. KALISS, N.: Immunological enhancement of tumor homografts: a review. Cancer Res. 18, 992 (1958).
22. HELLSTRÖM, K. E., HELLSTRÖM, I.: Immunological enhancement as studied by cell culture techniques. Ann. Rev. Microbiol. 24, 373 (1970).
23. HEPPNER, G. H.: Studies on serum-mediated inhibition of cellular immunity to spontanous mouse mammary tumors. Int. J. Cancer 4, 608 (1969).
24. SJÖGREN, H. O., HELLSTRÖM, I., BANSAL, S. C., HELLSTRÖM, K. E.: Suggestive evidence that the "blocking antibodies" of tumor-bearing individuals may be antigen-antibody complexes. Proc. nat. Acad. Sci. (Wash.) 68, 1372 (1971).
25. POLLACK, S., HEPPNER, G., BRAWN, R. J., NELSON, K.: Specific killing of tumor cells in vitro in the presence of normal lymphoid cells and sera from hosts immune to the tumor antigens. Int. J. Cancer, 9, 316 (1972).
26. WEISS, D. W., BONHAG, R. S., LESLIE, P.: Studies on the heterologous immunogenicity of a methanol-insoluble fraction of attenuated tubercle bacilli (BCG). J. exp. Med. 124, 1039 (1966).
27. STOLFI, R. L., MARTIN, D. S., FUGMANN, R. A.: Spontaneous murine mammary adenocarcinoma: Model system for evaluation of combined methods of therapy. Cancer Chemother. Rep. 55, 239 (1971).
28. CHECK, J. H., CHILDS, T. C., BRADY, L. W., DERASSE, A. R., FUSCALDO, K. E.: Protection against spontaneous mouse mammary adenocarcinoma by inoculation of heat-treated syngeneic mammary tumor cells. Int. J. Cancer 7, 403 (1971).
29. CALABRESI, P.: New techniques for measuring the effects of chemotherapeutic agents upon neoplastic and normal host cells. Vienna: Proc. 5th Int. Cong. of Chemotherapy 1967, p. 409.
30. HEPPNER, G. H., CALABRESI, P.: Suppression by cytosine arabinoside of serum blocking factors of cell-mediated immunity to syngeneic transplants of mouse mammary tumors. J. nat. Cancer Inst., 18, 1161 (1972).
31. MIKULSKA, Z. B., SMITH, C., ALEXANDER, P.: Evidence for an immunological reaction of the host directed against its own actively growing primary tumor. J. nat. Cancer Inst. 36, 29 (1966).
32. PREHN, R. T., MAIN, J. M.: Immunity to methylcholanthrene-induced sarcomas. J. nat. Cancer Inst. 18, 769 (1957).
33. HEPPNER, G. J.: In vitro studies on cell-mediated immunity following surgery in mice sensitized to syngeneic mammary tumors. Int. J. Cancer 9, 119 (1972).
34. MARTINEZ, C.: Effect of early thymectomy on development of mammary tumours in mice. Nature (Lond.) 203, 1188 (1964).
35. LAW, L. W.: Studies of thymic function with emphasis on the role of the thymus in oncogenesis. Cancer Res. 26, 551 (1966).
36. SAKAKURA, T., NISHIZUKA, Y.: Effect of thymectomy on mammary tumorigenesis, noduligenesis, and mammogenesis in the mouse. Gann 58, 441 (1967).
37. SQUARTINI, F., OLIVI, M., BOLIS, G. B.: Mouse strain and breeding stimulation as factors influencing the effect of thymectomy on mammary tumorigenesis. Cancer Res. 30, 2069 (1970).
38. YUNIS, E. J., MARTINEZ, C., SMITH, J., STUTMAN, O., GOOD, R. A.: Spontaneous mammary adenocarcinoma in mice: Influence of thymectomy and reconstitution with thymus grafts or spleen cells. Cancer Res. 29, 174 (1969).
39. HEPPNER, G. H.: Neonatal thymectomy and mouse mammary tumorigenesis. In: Immunity and Tolerance in Oncogenesis. Ed.: SEVERI, L. Perugia (Italy): University of Perugia 1970, p. 503.

40. Hellström, I., Hellström, K. E., Sjögren, H. O., Warner, G. A.: Demonstration of cell-mediated immunity to human neoplasms of various histological types. Int. J. Cancer 7, 1 (1971).
41. Andersen, V., Bjerrum, O., Bendixen, G., Schiødt, T., Dissing, T.: Effect of autologous mammary tumor extracts on human leucocyte migration in vitro. Int. J. Cancer 5, 357 (1970).
42. Black, M. M., Leis, H. P., Jr.: Cellular responses to autologous breast cancer tissue. Cancer (Philad.) 28, 263 (1971).
43. Moore, D. H., Charney, J., Kramarsky, B., Lasfargues, E. Y., Sarkar, N., Brennan, M. J., Burrows, J. H., Sirsat, S. M., Paymaster, J. C., Vaidya, A. B.: Search for a human breast cancer virus. Nature (Lond.) 229, 611 (1971).
44. Hellström, I., Sjögren, H. O., Warner, G., Hellström, K. E.: Blocking of cell-mediated tumor immunity by sera from patients with growing neoplasms. Int. J. Cancer 7, 226 (1971).
45. Hellström, I., Hellström, K. E., Sjögren, H. O., Warner, G. A.: Serum factors in tumor-free patients cancelling the blocking of cell-mediated tumor immunity. Int. J. Cancer 8, 185 (1971).

Cell Kinetics of Breast Cancer:
The Turnover of Nonproliferating Cells*

M. L. MENDELSOHN and L. A. DETHLEFSEN

The kinetic properties of growing tumors and of the involved normal tissues will probably continue for some time to be of major concern to biologists and therapists dealing with the cancer problem. To the extent that abnormal growth is the explicit manifestation of the malignant process, it is obviously relevant to learn as much as possible about the differences in growth dynamics of the tumor and the normal cell. In addition, all aspects of cancer therapy have a kinetic involvement. In radiotherapy the growth kinetics affect the rate of tumor shrinkage, the design of optimal fractionation, the estimation of numbers of tumor or normal cells at risk, and the use of combination or other treatment modifications to increase the therapeutic ratio of tumor to normal response. In chemotherapy the same problems repeat themselves and in addition the use of cycle-linked agents demands a keen insight into cell-cycle behavior and the noncycling cell. Finally in surgery as well as radiotherapy and chemotherapy, knowledge of the growth rate provides the framework within which one predicts and interprets the likely times of recurrence, the response to therapy, and the probability of cure.

The study of tumor kinetics has itself grown considerably since the advent of tritiated thymidine in 1957, and many excellent reviews attest to the progress that has been made (BASERGA, BRESCIANI, DENEKAMP, LALA, LAMERTON and STEEL, PERRY, SKIPPER, TUBIANA [1—8]). Nevertheless serious problems remain because of the poor resolution of the methods and their general unsuitability for clinical application. At present there is little the tumor kineticist can say to the clinician in the way of precise recommendations for optimizing treatment; but it is fair to say that the general insights into the mitotic process, the mechanism of action of drugs and radiation, the growth fraction, the natural history of tumor growth, and the comparative properties of tumor and normal tissues have had a major impact on the way clinical oncologists think about their patients. Where a decade ago a tumor was an exponentially growing mass of proliferating but otherwise nondescript cells, today the knowledgable oncologist visualizes cells in or out of a roughly known cell cycle, and he contrasts differentiating versus clonogenic cells, sensitive versus resistant cells, young tumors versus old tumors, and so on. These concepts or models of cancer growth are still

* This work was supported in part by USPHS Grant 5 K06 CA18540, 5 K04 CA-42,352, 5 R01 CA03896 and FR 15; and by the Atomic Energy Commission (COO-3087-1).

Sincere appreciation in the performance of these experiments is expressed to WILLIAM JENKINS, REBA RILEY, JOSEPH HOGG, and STEVEN L. MENDELSOHN

naive and inadequate and have only barely been fitted to human data, but they begin to describe tumors in general and some tumors in particular, and they offer a foundation for future study.

A Kinetic Model and Its Application to Solid Tumors

Our current view of a minimal model for solid tumors is shown in Fig. 1. The tumor cells fall into three categories: P, the proliferating cells; Q, the nonproliferating cells; and L, the cells that have been lost due to cell death or migration. The P cells are the driving force for tumor growth and their net effect depends on the duration of their cell cycle and their rates of conversion to Q and L cells. The actual

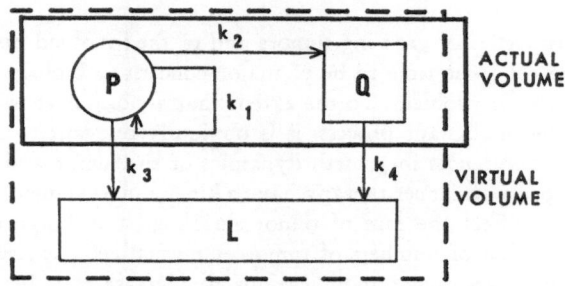

Fig. 1. Simplified Kinetic Model of Tumor Growth. The model contains three homogeneous compartments of cells: P, the proliferating cells; Q, the nonproliferating cells; and L, the cells that are lost by migration or death. The four rate constants, k_1 to k_4, describe the net flow between compartments; but k_2 is the only one that could conceivably involve flow in both directions. The virtual volume is what would exist if L cells maintained their integrity and hence is a representation of the potential growth of the tumor

cellular volume of the tumor is $P + Q$, and the growth fraction or proportion of proliferating cells is $P/(P+Q)$. The effect of cell loss can be imagined in terms of a virtual cellular volume which contains the actual cellular volume plus the dead, dying and otherwise departed L cells. The growth rate of $P + Q + L$ is the virtual cellular growth rate or production rate, and is equivalent to the potential cellular growth rate of Steel. Associated with the actual and virtual cellular volumes, there are corresponding total volumes which include the acellular contents of the tumor (e. g., the necrotic regions, cysts, alveolar and ductular spaces, and vascular space).

The cyclic proliferative properties of the P cells can be studied by the FLM (fraction of labeled mitoses) method of Quastler and Sherman, as modified by one of the recent mathematical fitting procedures for extracting the kinetic parameters (STEEL and HANES; MACDONALD; and TAKAHASHI, HOGG and MENDELSOHN [10—12]). Pulse labeling with specific radioactive precursors of DNA is followed by the removal and fixation of tumors or tumors samples at selected times, autoradiography, and identification of the fraction of labeled mitotic cells. In carefully done experiments this provides estimates for the mean and distribution of cell cycle times, as well as for a variety of other parameters of the cell cycle.

The expected labeling index of the P cells is a function of time after labeling and of the position and relative duration of the DNA synthetic phase of the cell cycle.

Initially the Q cells do not label, and hence the labeling index of the tumor as a whole is a combination of the expected P cell labeling index and the proportion of Q cells in the population. By measuring the observed labeling index and either calculating or measuring the expected P cell labeling index, it is possible to estimate the growth fraction (MENDELSOHN [13]; STEEL [14]).

The growth fraction and the mean cell cycle time determine how fast the tumor should grow. When this potential cellular growth rate is compared to the observed volumetric growth rate of the tumor, the difference is ascribable to the rate of cell loss (STEEL [14]; MENDELSOHN [15]). STEEL, ADAMS and BARRETT [16], raised the possibility that cell loss might reflect an aging process peculiar to the Q cells, but in general the kinetic literature assumes cell loss to be a combined exponential property of the entire tumor population.

The Turnover Time of Q Cells

Q cells are immune to the cycle-linked effects of chemotherapy (and perhaps of radiotherapy) and as long as they remain viable and nonproliferative they are frustratingly out of reach of many therapeutic approaches. Thus it seemed worthwhile to us to push the resolution of kinetic analysis to the point where the turnover time of Q cells could be estimated. This in effect provides the partitioning of cell loss between the P and Q compartments and allows estimates of the four rate constants in Fig. 1 as well as the magnitudes of the three compartments.

The mathematical description of Q cell turnover (or for that matter of any of the kinetic phenomena we have presented) is inappropriate here, but enough of the principle of the method will be given to allow the reader to understand and evaluate the data that are to follow.

The key to following the behavior of Q cells is the change of the tumor labeling index with time. Immediately after pulse-labeling, a proportion of P cells is labeled and all of the Q cells are unlabeled. As the tumor grows, the P cells multiply, maintain a slightly oscillating but more-or-less constant labeling index, and progressively populate the Q and L compartments. Thus the labeling index of the Q cells begins at zero, but steadily increases toward the P cell labeling index as the originally unlabeled and nongrowing Q cells are diluted by new Q cells or are lost by attrition. The labeling index of the tumor as a whole is a weighted average of the indices of the P and Q cells, and hence it too gradually asymptotes toward the P cell value.

If the labeling index of the P cells is measured (for example, by measuring the fraction of labeled mitoses after damping of the FLM curve), or better still, if an expected labeling index, $LI_{exp}(t)$, is computed from the cell cycle parameters of the proliferating cells, then

$$\frac{Q_0(t)}{P(t)+Q(t)} = 1 - \frac{LI_{obs}(t)}{LI_{exp}(t)}$$

or in other words, at time t, the Q_0 or initially unlabeled Q cells can be estimated as a proportion of total cells by using a function of the $LI_{exp}(t)$ and the observed labeling index for the tumor as a whole, $LI_{obs}(t)$.

The effect of three contrasting types of Q cell turnover illustrates how the labeling indices behave. Consider first a tumor with no cell loss and a constant growth fraction. The P and Q cells increase at the same relative growth rate, as do $P+Q$ or

tumor cell volume and $V_a(t)$ the actual volume (assuming a constant fraction of the tumor is tumor cells). The number of Q_0 cells remains constant but the proportion, $Q_0/(P+Q)$, will decrease with the growth of the denominator. Thus the change in

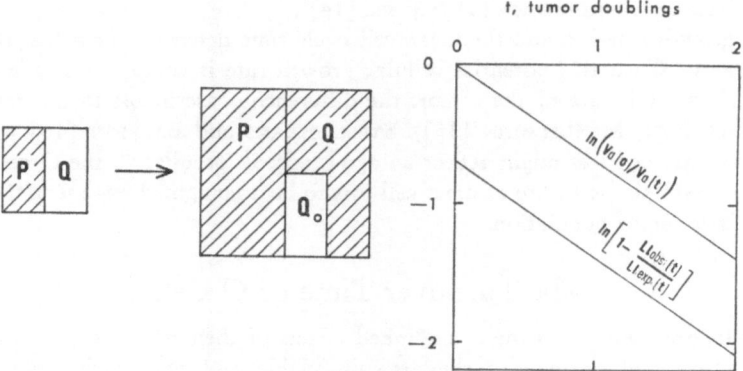

Fig. 2. Model 1—no loss of Q cells. The progressive dilution of unlabeled Q_0 cells by labeled P and Q cells results in an observed labeling index, $LI_{obs}(t)$, that rises toward the expected labeling index of P cells, $LI_{exp}(t)$, as a function of actual volume, $V_a(t)$. Thus the slope of $\ln[1-LI_{obs}(t)/LI_{exp}(t)]$ is identical to the slope of $\ln[V_a(0)/V_a(t)]$. In the diagram the areas represent compartment size and the shading refers to cells with the expected labeling index. The smaller diagram is at the moment of labeling with a DNA precursor, and the larger diagram is two doubling times later when the actual volume has increased fourfold. Since there is no cell loss the virtual and actual volumes are identical. The growth fraction is 0.5. The ordinates in this graph and in Figs. 3, 4, and 8—10 are given along side the lines

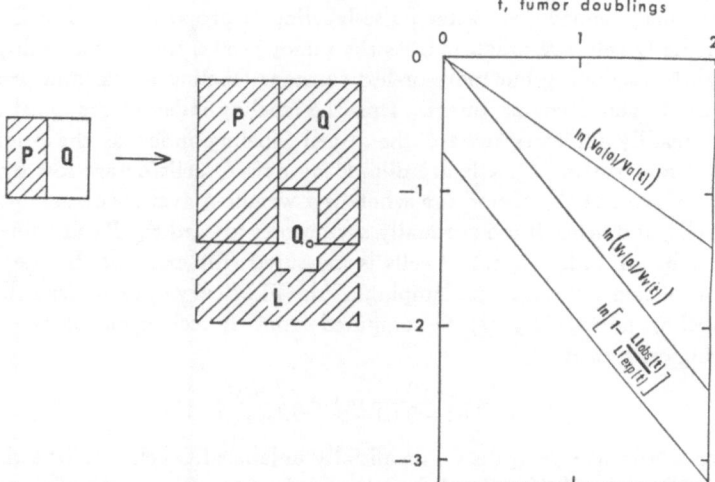

Fig. 3. Model 2—equivalent loss of P and Q cells. Cumulative cell loss over the two doubling times has been added to the larger diagram and corresponds to the virtual growth line shown in the graph as $\ln[V_v(0)/V_v(t)]$. The diagram also shows the Q_0 cells that are lost by attrition. Now the decay of the proportion of residual Q_0 cells is equivalent to dilution by the virtual volume and hence $\ln[1-LI_{obs}(t)/LI_{exp}(t)]$ has the same slope as $\ln[V_v(0)/V_v(t)]$

$1 - LI_{obs}(t)/LI_{exp}(t)$ will also mirror the change in volume. This is shown diagrammatically in Fig. 2 for an exponentially growing tumor, in which case both $\ln[1 - LI_{obs}(t)/LI_{exp}(t)]$ and $\ln[V_a(0)/V_a(t)]$ should be linear functions of time and should have identical slopes. The same relationships will hold if cell death is present but is limited to P cells.

Consider next a tumor in which cell death is independent of the proliferative status of the cells and hence in which P and Q cells have an equal probability of dying. Now in addition to dilution of the Q_0 cells, some Q_0 cells will be lost to the L compartment. The overall effect is equivalent to dilution based on $V_v(t)$ the virtual volume and $\ln[1 - LI_{obs}(t)/LI_{exp}(t)]$ will now have the same slope as $\ln[V_v(0)/V_v(t)]$. This is shown in Fig. 3.

Finally there is the possibility of selective loss of only Q cells. In this situation the slope of $\ln[1 - LI_{obs}(t)/LI_{exp}(t)]$ is steeper than the slopes attributable to either actual or virtual volume. This is shown in Fig. 4.

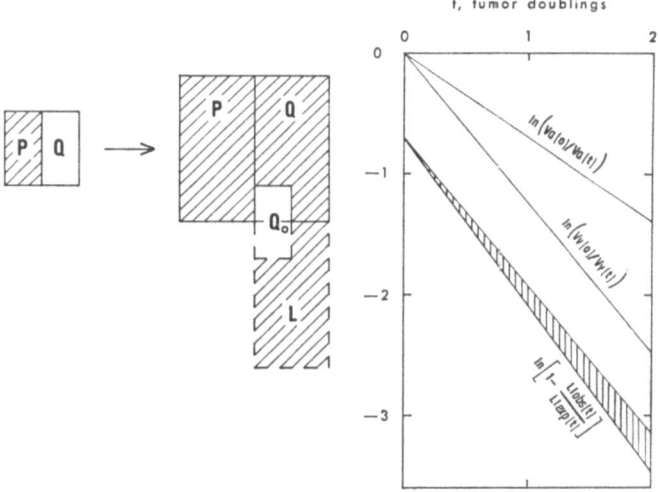

Fig. 4. Model 3—preferential loss of Q cells. The same conditions prevail except that now cell loss is limited to Q cells. This increases the attrition rate of Q_0 cells with the result that $\ln[1 - LI_{obs}(t)/LI_{exp}(t)]$ has a steeper slope than $\ln[V_v(0)/V_v(t)]$. The shaded area on the graph shows the full range of response, from no bias against Q cells to the present case of total bias. To explain even more rapid decay of the proportion of Q_0 cells, it is necessary to invoke either a fixed comparatively short life span of Q cells or a steeply increasing risk of dying with age of Q cells

Application to Mouse Mammary Tumors

The turnover of nonproliferating cells has been studied in three experimental tumor lines carried in isogenic C3H mice. These lines are part of a long-term study of serial transplantation with forced selection for specific growth characteristics (DETHLEFSEN and MENDELSOHN [21]). The Slow Line began as a "spontaneous" C3H mammary tumor. By appropriate selection at each transplant generation, the growth rate has been held stable from the eighth through the 35th generation. The line was in

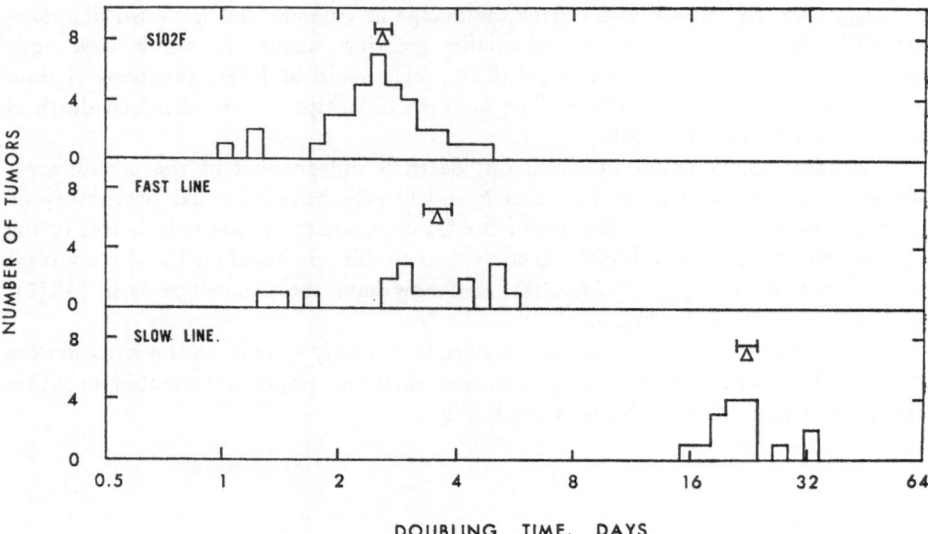

Fig. 5. The distribution of estimated tumor doubling time. As a general rule these mammary tumors do not grow exponentially but follow an approximately cube-root growth curve. For each tumor, a three-parameter growth curve was fitted to the volumetric measurements, and then the computed growth rates during the short interval between labeling and fixation were used to calculate the exponential doubling time. The mean doubling time and its standard error is shown for each line

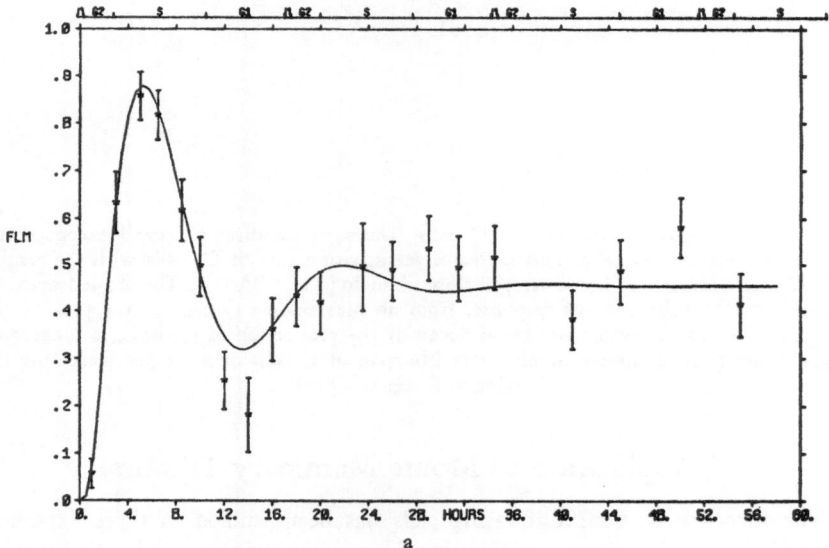

Fig. 6. a—c FLM data and computer fitted FLM curves. The x's are means of FLM values for all tumors fixed at the same time. The bars represent the 95% confidence limits of binomial counting error. The cell cycle parameters of these best-fitting curves are given in the table. Rapidly damped FLM curves such as these are typical of solid tumors with their highly variable cell cycle times. a S 102 F, b fast, c slow

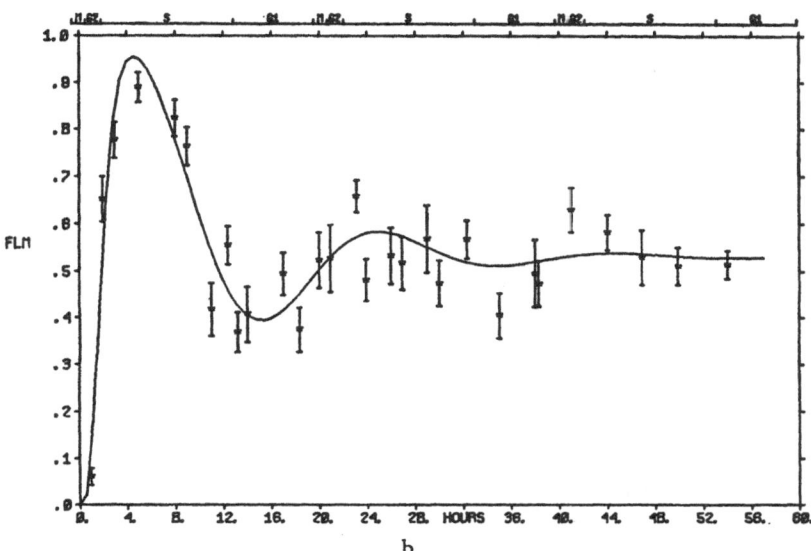

b

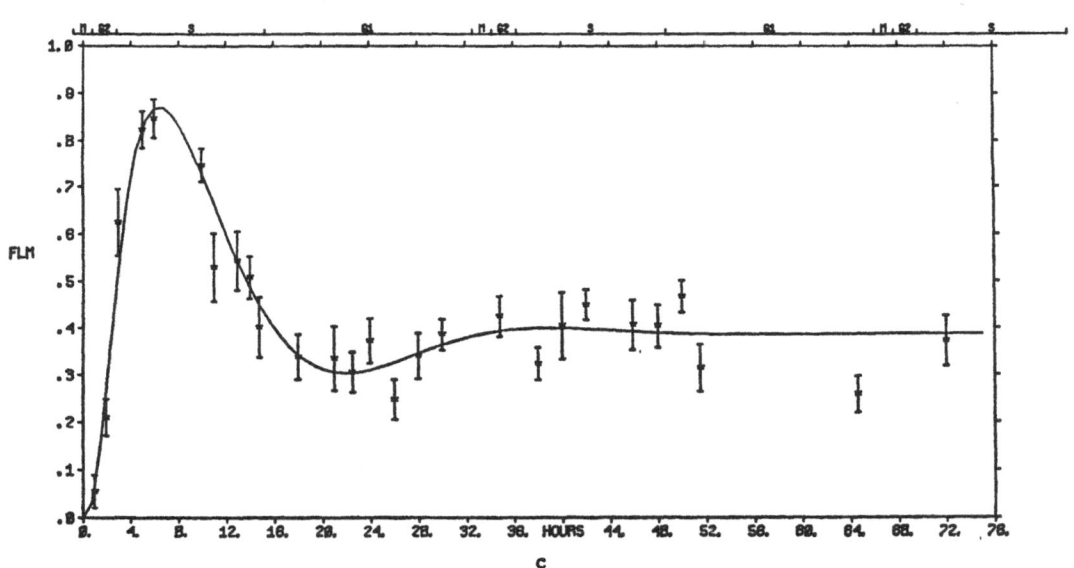

c

its fifth generation when this study was done, at which time the tumors were at 80%
of their asymptotic growth rate and were slowly accelerating. The Fast Line derives
from another "spontaneous" C3H mammary tumor and a stable growth rate has been
maintained from the 17th to the 65th generation. During the tenth and 11th generation when this study was done, this line was also within 80% of its asymptotic value
and was slowly increasing its growth rate. The S102F Line had a similar origin from
yet another "spontaneous" tumor. For the first 15 generations its growth rate was
enhanced by deliberately selecting the fastest transplant in each generation for further

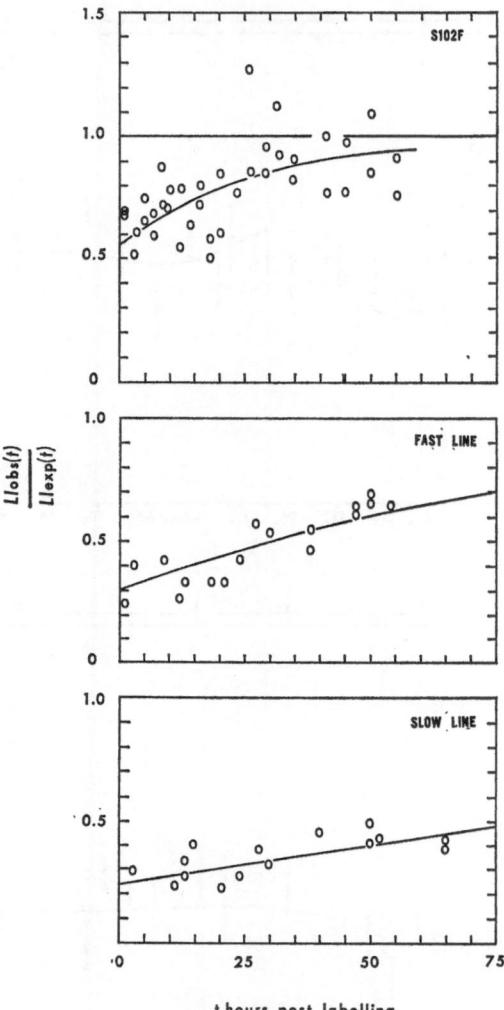

Fig. 7. The ratio of observed to expected labeling index for the three tumor lines. The expected labeling index, $LI_{exp}(t)$, is computed from the fitted FLM curve and is the expected value as a function of time for P cells and their descendants. The fitted curves are a translation of the lines shown in Figs. 8—10. The growth fraction is $LI_{obs}(0)/LI_{exp}(0)$ and hence is the intersection of each curve with the y axis

propagation. From the 15th to the 54th generation the growth rate has been stabilized and the present study was done on tumors from the 19th generation.

Volumetric growth was followed serially by caliper measurements in three dimensions. Computer fits of the data for each tumor were made to determine the individual growth rates, incremental growth, and calculated doubling time during the labeling experiment (DETHLEFSEN, PREWITT and MENDELSOHN [17]). The distribution of doubling times for the entire experiment is summarized in Fig. 5.

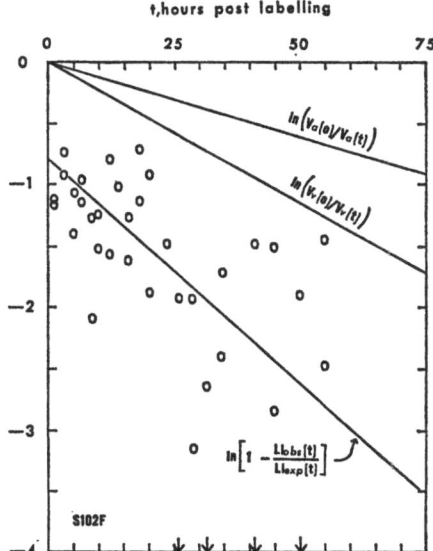

Fig. 8. The changing proportion of Q_0 cells in S102F tumors. The logarithmically transformed data of labeling indices and the mean responses of actual and virtual volumes for these tumors are shown. In spite of the wide scatter in the data, the slope of $\ln [1-LI_{obs}(t)/LI_{exp}(t)]$ line is steeper than either of the others, indicating that this is closest to a Model 3 situation with selective loss of Q cells. The arrows refer to the four tumors in which the ratio of observed to expected labeling index was one or greater

The S102F series was labeled with tritiated 5-iodo-2'-deoxyuridine and tritiated thymidine was used for the Slow and Fast lines. Two or more tumors were usually fixed at each experimental time. Autoradiographs were exposed in geometric progression and the optimum exposure was then selected retrospectively for each tumor. The bulk of counts were done blind, using several observers and counting a minimum of 100 and usually over 200 mitoses per specimen. The FLM curves were fit by the method of TAKAHASHI, HOGG and MENDELSOHN [12], including a recent modification of the program to give the expected value of the labeling index of P cells as a function of time after labeling. Labeling indices were based on counts of 200 or more labeled cells, and particular attention was paid to obtain uniform sampling over the entire population of intact cells.

Table

Cell cycle parameters					
T_i, hours (CV_i, %)					Standard deviation from regression, FLM units
Line	G_1	S	G_2	M	C	
S102F	6.50 (71)	7.69 (45)	2.47 (58)	0.55 (58)	17.22 (34)	0.069
Fast	6.71 (45)	10.97 (50)	1.34 (58)	1.10 (58)	20.13 (32)	0.075
Slow	17.34 (71)	12.48 (58)	2.05 (71)	1.60 (71)	33.46 (43)	0.063

Fig. 6 shows the FLM data and the computer fitted FLM curves, and the table summarizes the cell cycle parameters extracted from the three tumor lines. The ratio of observed to expected labeling indices are shown in Fig. 7, and Figs. 8—10 give $\ln[1-LI_{obs}(t)/LI_{exp}(t)]$, as well as the measured $\ln[V_a(0)/V_a(t)]$ and the calculated $\ln[V_v(0)/V_v(t)]$ for each tumor line.

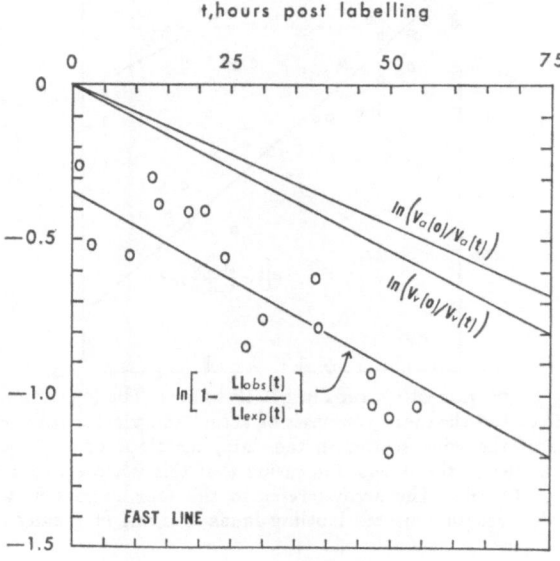

Fig. 9. The changing proportion of Q_0 cells in Fast Line tumors. The similarity of slope of the actual and virtual volumes indicates a low rate of cell loss, and again $\ln[1-LI_{obs}(t)/LI_{exp}(t)]$ is the steepest response of the three. Hence these tumors also show selective loss of Q cells

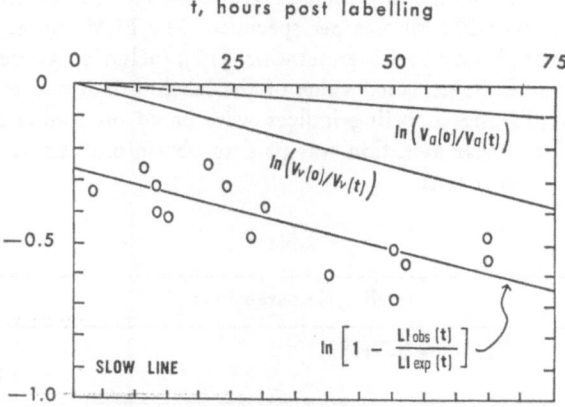

Fig. 10. The changing proportion of Q_0 cells in Slow Line tumors. Cell loss is extensive, as indicated by the difference in slopes of actual and virtual volumes. Unlike the other tumors, Slow Line tumors show a slope for $\ln[1-LI_{obs}(t)/LI_{exp}(t)]$ that is identical to the slope for $\ln[V_v(0)/V_v(t)]$. Hence in this case loss is equally likely in the P and Q compartments

S102F has a relative volumetric growth rate of 28.8% per day and is the fastest growing of the three tumor lines. It also has the shortest cell cycle time, with a mean of 17.2 hours. Its labeling indices are the most extensive and probably the least ambiguous of the three sets, but there is a large amount of scattering of the data points as

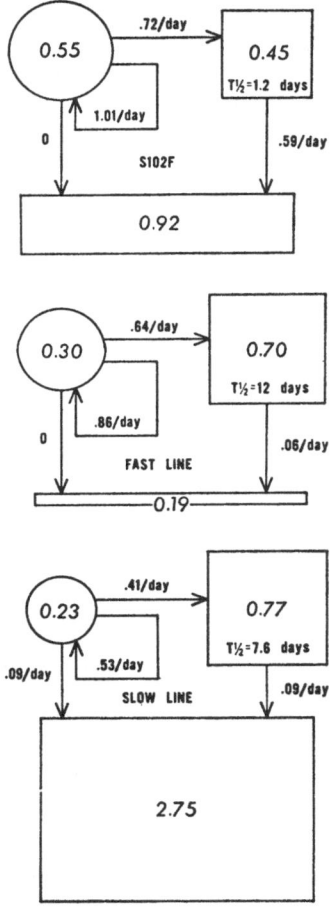

Fig. 11. The estimated compartment sizes and rate constants for the three tumor lines. Compartment sizes are drawn to scale and are given as a proportion of $P+Q$. The feedback constant, k_1, of the P compartment is the computed growth constant provided by the FLM analysis. It is approximated by ln 2 divided by the mean cell cycle time, but is actually slightly larger because of the effects of the skewed distribution of cell cycle times used in the Takahashi model. The $T^{1/2}$ is the estimated half time of turnover of the Q compartment

shown in Figs. 7 and 8. Iterative fitting by hand indicates that the first two death models are incompatible with the data. In fact, the fit to model three (i. e., selective death in the Q compartment) satisfies the data only when the death rates in Q account for essentially all cell loss in the tumor. The definitive rate constants and the compartment sizes are shown in Fig. 11. One notes that the growth fraction is 0.55, the relative production rate is 55% of tumor cells per day, the loss rate is 27% per day, and the Q cells turnover with a half time of 1.2 days .

The Fast Line has a relative growth rate of 21.6% of volume per day and its cell cycle time averages 20.1 hours. The relative production rate is 25.6% per day, and because this value is so similar to the relative volumetric growth rate, this tumor shows very little cell loss (4.0% per day). Judging from the labeling indices in Figs. 7 and 9, this tumor is also compatible with the third model and again the loss of Q cells accounts for all cell loss. However in this case the turnover of Q cells is considerably slower, giving a half time of 12 days. The growth fraction is 0.23.

The Slow Line has a relative volumetric growth rate of 3.3% of volume per day and a mean cell cycle of 33.5 hours. The relative production rate is 12.4% per day and hence cell loss amounts to 9.1% per day. In contrast to the other two lines, the Slow Line is best approximated by the second model in which loss is equally probable for P and Q cells. The resulting turnover time of Q cells is 7.6 days and the Growth Fraction is 0.23.

Interpretation

These results involve a convolution of several techniques, each of which is vulnerable to noise, experimental bias, and over-simplification of what is likely to be the reality of tumor growth. Thus there is good reason to avoid over-reliance on the final details, at least until the values can be confirmed by independent methods or some sort of global error analysis can be done. Our impression is that growth rates of individual tumors are reliable to well within 10%, and that the cell cycle parameters have coefficients of variation of estimation of 5 to 10%. However we are unable to put concrete estimates of error on the assumption of exponential behavior in Figs. 8 to 10, on the scatter of the labeling indices, and on such confounding influences as reutilization of label and heterogeneity of the cell populations. For the moment the experiment is best viewed as a crude approximation sitting right at the feasible limit of kinetic analysis of such experimental systems. Amongst other things, this is a rather pessimistic implication for the parallel development with human tumors. If this is the best we can do with a well behaved and large homogeneous series of transplanted small animal tumors, what can possibly be expected from the human situation in which a dozen or so biopsies of a single neoplasm is already a heroic experiment?

The view that a tumor can be modeled effectively by three homogeneous populations of cells is patently oversimplified. A more realistic but presently intractable series of models would include many more components. There would be multiple subpopulations of P, Q and L cells representing genetically divergent clones, neoplastic progression, and different pathways of differentiation within the tumor. These subpopulations would change as a function of time, of tumor size, and of therapy. One or more of them would represent the cells that had retained clonogenic capacity and hence would describe the kinetics of the particular cells whose survival decides whether or not a tumor is to be cured. For the radiotherapist there would be subdivisions into oxygenated and hypoxic cells, and perhaps into cells with varying capacity for repair of sublethal injury. For the chemotherapist a similar partitioning would be based on the pharmacologic parameters that affect accessibility and inherent metabolic sensitivity to drug (HALL [19]). A complete model would also include the kinetics of relevant stromal elements and in particular the growth properties of tumor vasculature (TANNOCK and HAYASHI [22]).

In spite of the noisy measurements and the oversimplified interpretation, the results we have obtained make reasonable sense in terms of what little is known about the biology of our three tumor types. For some years we have been aware of the heterogeneous behavior of growth and death in the Slow Line (MENDELSOHN, DETH-LEFSEN and JENKINS [20]). This is clearly a tumor in which cell death can be due to the risks of cell division, to differentiation into highly organized ducts, and to gross necrosis of entire tissue regions. Thus one would expect cell loss from both the P and Q compartments, although not necessarily equiprobable loss from each. The histology of S102F tumors is considerably simpler than that of the Slow Line. The S102F tumors consist of highly repetitious, apparently ductular structures in which the cell linings are only one or two cells thick. Free cells in various stages of degen-eration are seen within the ductules, and the entire process is consistent with a proliferating basal layer, an incomplete and short-lived differentiating layer, and cell loss into the lumen. The Fast Line is microscopically organized into lobules of poorly differentiated acini. The tumor has little stroma, is soft and almost semi-fluid, and has no gross necrosis.

The two indications of selective loss of Q cells should be encouraging to the therapist. Given the existence of some known rate of cell loss, then the best one can hope for is that all of the loss comes from the otherwise unreachable Q cells. Obviously one cannot generalize from only two examples, and perhaps the over-riding point is that there is remarkably little evidence of conformity in these three mammary tumors of common genetic and etiologic origin. The growth rates, cell cycles, growth fractions, and all other kinetic parameters vary greatly, as do the gross and microscopic appearances. Is it reasonable, then, to expect conformity of human tumors, or is every neoplasm likely to be kinetically unique? Our earlier experience with kinetic analysis of the "spontaneous" C3H mammary tumor pointed more to commonness than the uniqueness (MENDELSOHN [15]), and the few human tumors that have been studied seem to support this view (see TUBIANA for review). Perhaps the divergence of the three tumor lines is a result of the many generations of transplantation and hence is an overly pessimistic view of the behavior of the autochthonous tumor.

The prospects that kinetic analysis will become part of the work-up of the cancer patient remains very remote. For what it is worth, the extra step we have added in this paper does not complicate the analysis since our method requires only the repeated estimation of the labeling index after pulse labeling and hence one can use the same specimens one would obtain for a labeled mitosis curve. However, the latter is already a prohibitive procedure, requiring multiple samples, much labor, and an interval of a month or so for exposure of the autoradiographs. If we kineticists are to help it will not be by pushing these methods into the clinic, but rather by dis-covering more tractable procedures or by using our models and experimental tumor systems to gain broad insights into the therapeutic process. Given the framework of a therapeutic rational, the clinical therapist should be able to converge more rapidly toward optimal strategies, but the clinical phases of the optimization process—at least from the kinetic viewpoint—are likely to remain empirical for some time to come.

References

1. Baserga, R., Wiebel, F.: The cell cycle of mammalian cells. Int. Rev. exp. Path. 7, 1 (1969).
2. Bresciani, F.: Cell proliferation in cancer. Europ. J. Cancer 4, 343 (1968).
3. Denekamp, J.: The cellular proliferation kinetics of animal tumours. Cancer Res. 30, 393 (1970).
4. Lala, P. K.: Studies on tumor cell population kinetics. In: Methods in Cancer Research, vol. 6. New York: Academic Press 1971, p. 3.
5. Lamerton, L. F., Steel, G. G.: Cell population kinetics in normal and malignant tissues. In: Progress in Biophysics and Molecular Biology. Pergamon Press 1968, p. 247.
6. Perry, S.: Human tumor cell kinetics. Lecture Series. Nat. Cancer Inst. Monograph No. 30 (1969).
7. Skipper, H. E.: Cancer chemotherapy is many things. G.H.A. Clowes Memorial Lecture. Cancer Res. 31, 1173 (1971).
8. Tubiana, M.: The kinetics of tumour cell proliferation and radiotherapy. Brit. J. Radiol. 44, 325 (1971).
9. Quastler, H., Sherman, F. G.: Cell population kinetics in the intestinal epithelium of the mouse. Exp. Cell Res. 17, 240 (1959).
10. Macdonald, P. D. M.: Statistical inference from the fraction labelled mitoses curve. Biometrika 57, 489 (1970).
11. Steel, G. G., Hanes, S.: The technique of labelled mitoses: analysis by automatic curve-fitting. Cell & Tissue Kinetics 4, 93 (1971).
12. Takahashi, M., Hogg, J. D., Mendelsohn, M. L.: The automatic analysis of FLM curves. Cell & Tissue Kinetics 4, 505 (1971).
13. Mendelsohn, M. L.: Autoradiographic analysis of cell proliferation in spontaneous breast cancer of C3H mouse III. The growth fraction. J. nat. Cancer Inst. 28, 1015 (1962).
14. Steel, G. G.: Cell loss from experimental tumours. Cell & Tissue Kinetics 1, 193 (1968).
15. Mendelsohn, M. L.: The kinetics of tumor cell proliferation. In: Cellular Radiation Biology. Baltimore: Williams & Wilkins 1965, p. 498.
16. Steel, G. G., Adams, K., Barrett, J. C.: Analysis of the cell population kinetics of transplanted tumours of widely-differing growth rate. Brit. J. Cancer 20, 784 (1966).
17. Dethlefsen, L. A., Prewitt, J. M. S., Mendelsohn, M. L.: Analysis of tumor growth curves. J. nat. Cancer Inst. 40, 389 (1968).
18. Takahashi, M.: Theoretical basis for cell cycle analysis II. Further studies on labelled mitosis wave method. J. theor. Biol. 18, 195 (1968).
19. Hall, T. C.: Limited role of cell kinetics in clinical cancer chemotherapy. In: Prediction of Response in Cancer Therapy. Nat. Cancer Inst. Monogr. 34, 15 (1971).
20. Mendelsohn, M. L., Dethlefsen, L. A., Jenkins, W. H.: In: Time and Dose Relationships in Radiation Biology as Applied to Radiotherapy. NCI-AEC Conference. Carmel, California, BNL-50203. Upton. New York: Brookhaven Nat. Lab. Associated Universities Inc., 1969, p. 149.
21. Dethlefsen, L. A., Mendelsohn, M. L.: The effects of selection and passage on the volumetric growth rate of mouse mammary tumors. Manuscript in preparation.
22. Tannock, I. F., Hayashi, S.: The proliferation of capillary endothelial cells. Cancer Res. 32, 77 (1972).

Breast Cancer Survival Over Three Decades

M. H. MYERS

Introduction

It is important to examine survival in the general run of breast cancer patients so that we can determine to what extent treatment methods are accomplishing what we would like to see—namely that the methods currently employed are curing at least some patients. Data are presented covering the time period 1940—1969 that have been accumulated by the End Results Group which is sponsored by the National Cancer Institute.

The End Results Group was created in 1956 for the purpose of pulling together in a systematic fashion, data on cancer patient survival so that new advances in therapeutic methods could be evaluated. The End Results Group is now made up of 6 hospital tumor registries associated with medical schools (the University of Chicago Clinics is one of these registries) and three centralized tumor registries. Thus the data that are presented come to the National Cancer Institute from over 100 hospitals representing the gamut from small community hospitals to large general hospitals and university medical centers.

In order to set the stage for discussions of survival, consider the following facts about breast cancer:

1. Connecticut data reported by CUTLER, CHRISTINE and BARCLAY [1] show that breast cancer incidence has been on the increase since the 1940's from 55 per 100,000 in 1940—44 to 72 per 100,000 in 1965—68. These authors also observed an increase in incidence for the population of Saskatchewan, Canada from 52 per 100,000 in 1950—52 to 66 per 100,000 in 1967—69. The Connecticut figure for 1965—68 of 72 per 100,000 is consistent with the reported figure for 1969 at 74 per 100,000 from the Third National Cancer Survey [2].

2. Breast cancer accounts for approximately one fourth of the malignancies that occur in women.

Stage and Treatment Distribution

A total of over 63,000 breast cancer cases have been assembled by the End Results Group during the period 1940—1969. Table 1 shows that over this period of time the percent of breast cancers diagnosed while localized has increased slightly, but seems to have reached a plateau during the 1960's at 46 to 47%. Throughout the thirty year period slightly over 40% of breast cancer patients were diagnosed in the

Table 1. Breast cancer stage distribution (%)

	Year of diagnosis			
	1940—49	1950—59	1960—64	1965—69
No. of patients	12,184	22,105	13,828	14,911
Percent				
localized	38	42	46	47
regional	43	41	42	41
distant	14	13	10	10
other	5	4	2	2

Table 2. Breast cancer treatment distribution for localized cases (%)

	Year of diagnosis			
	1940—49	1950—59	1960—64	1965—69
No. of patients	4,998	10,431	7,084	6,956
Percent treated by surgery:				
Alone	78	85	77	78
With radiation	13	10	11	14
With chemo./horm.	0	1	6	5
Total surgery	91	96	94	97

Table 3. Breast cancer treatment distribution for regional cases (%)

	Year of diagnosis			
	1940—49	1950—59	1960—64	1965—69
No. of patients	5,804	10,221	6,574	6,160
Percent treated by surgery:				
Alone	56	57	42	36
With radiation	27	30	38	46
With chemo./horm.	0	2	6	5
With radiation and chemo./horm.	1	2	6	7
Total surgery	86	93	96	94

regional stage while the percent with distant involvement has decreased from 14 to 10%.

Table 2 gives the treatment patterns for patients with localized breast cancer. It is perhaps no surprise that surgery is used in over 90% of patients with localized disease and has increased to a high of 97% for patients diagnosed during 1965—69. Radiation is being used as an adjunct to surgery in slightly over 10% of these patients.

For breast cancer patients with disease spread to regional areas, there has been an increase in the use of radiation as an adjunct to surgery from 28% in 1940—49 to 53% in 1965—69 (Table 3). During the 1960's 12% of regional patients received chemotherapy or hormones in addition to surgery.

Survival

The survival data are in terms of the relative survival rate which is by definition the ratio of the observed proportion surviving to the expected proportion for women of similar age in the general population [3]. Fig. 1 shows for all stages of breast cancer that there was improvement in survival from the 1940's to 1960—64 but data available for patients diagnosed during 1965—69 indicate no further improvement. Notice that for the time periods for which long follow-up is available, the curves continue to have a downward slope even after 15 to 20 years. If breast cancer patients had achieved survival equivalent to that in the general population (this would be "cure" in a statistical sense) the survival curves would have become parallel to the horizontal axis.

BREAST CANCER-ALL STAGES: 1940-1969

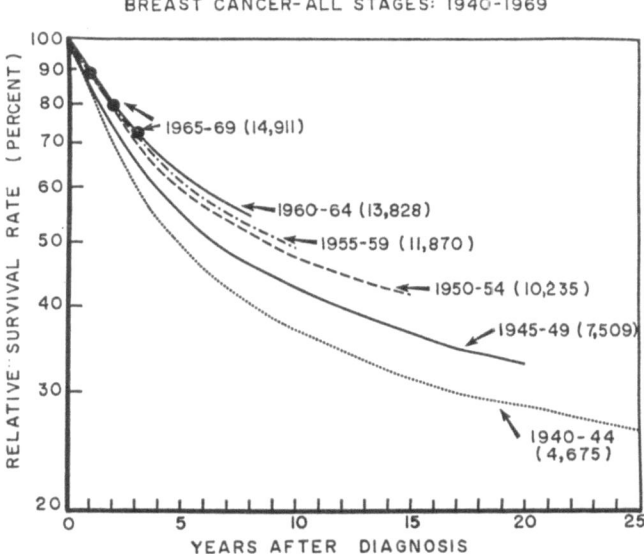

Fig. 1. Relative survival for female breast cancer patients by calendar period of diagnosis: *all stages*. The number of patients in each cohort is in parenthesis

Survival for patients with localized disease is at a reasonably high level and improved from the 1940's to the early 1950's but has been at approximately the same level since that time (Fig. 2). Again, even for localized disease survival after 15 years of follow-up does not reach that expected of similar patients in the general population.

Fig. 3 indicates that for patients with regional involvement the survival picture has been improving from the 1940's through the latter half of the 1950's.

Table 4 presents a summary of the survival results in terms of 3 and 5-year relative survival rates. The 5-year projections for 1965—69 are based on the assumption that survival subsequent to 3-years for which follow-up was available would be no worse than that observed for patients diagnosed during 1960—64.

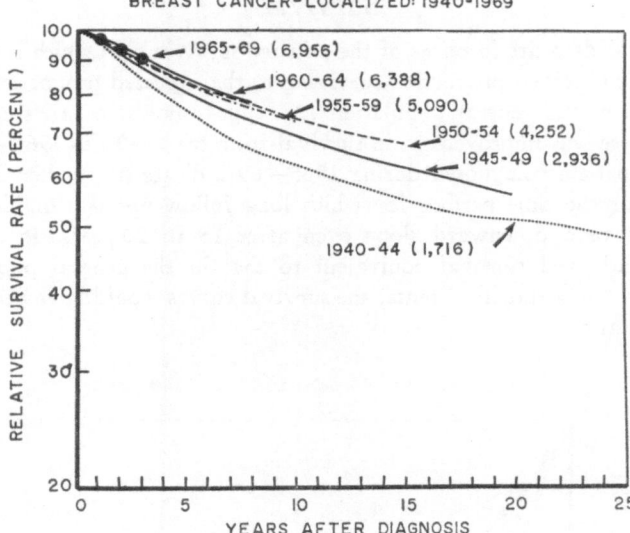

Fig. 2. Relative survival for female breast cancer patients by calendar period of diagnosis: *localized*. The number of patients in each cohort is in parenthesis

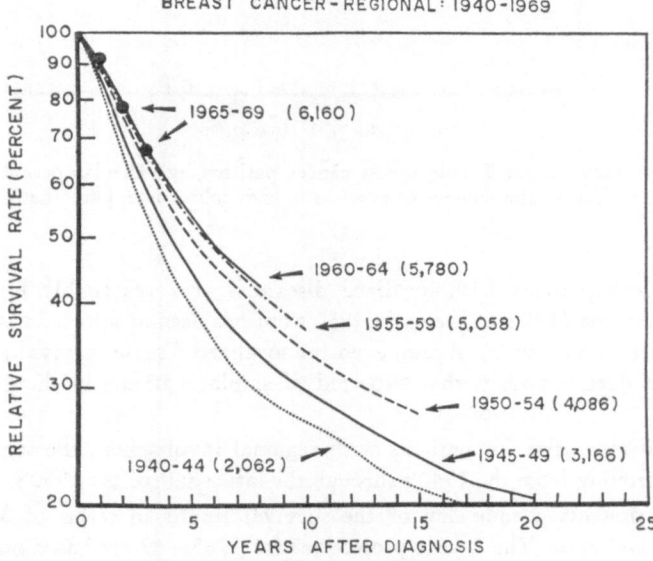

Fig. 3. Relative survival for female breast cancer patients by calendar period of diagnosis: *regional*. The number of patients in each cohort is in parenthesis

Table 4. Survival by stage: 3 and 5-year relative survival rates (%)

Stage	Year of diagnosis			
	1940—49	1950—59	1960—64	1965—69
All stages				
3-year	63	71	73	72
5-year	53	60	63	62 [a]
Localized				
3-year	86	89	91	91
5-year	78	83	84	83 [a]
Regional				
3-year	56	65	67	68
5-year	42	51	53	54 [a]
Distant				
3-year	22	27	14	15
5-year	15	17	7	8 [a]

[a] These projections are based on the assumption that survival subsequent to 3 years is no worse than that for patients diagnosed during 1960—64.

Discussion

We must keep in mind that 50% or more of breast cancer patients are 45—64 years of age at diagnosis and that a period of 15 to 20 years of follow-up may reduce the significance of the fact that "cure" is not achieved in a statistical sense. Recurring or metastatic breast cancer is still not pleasant to look forward to after having already escaped the risk for such an extended period of time.

The data presented have shown some improvement in survival over time although this trend does not extend to the most recent time period for which data are available. The survival picture for all breast cancer patients as a group could be improved by diagnosing a higher percentage of patients while the cancer is localized. This too seems to have stabilized unless some of the newer diagnostic techniques are made available to the general population. Apparently reduction of the excess risk of dying of breast cancer even for localized disease awaits some new therapeutic methods.

References

1. CUTLER, S. J., CHRISTINE, B., BARCLAY, T. H. C.: Increasing Incidence and Decreasing Mortality Rates for Breast Cancer. Cancer (Philad.) 28, 1376—1380 (1971).
2. Preliminary Report, Third National Cancer Survey, 1969 Incidence. DHEW Publication No. (NIH) 72—128 (1971).
3. AXTELL, L. M.: Computing Survival Rates for Chronic Disease Patients. A Simple Procedure. J. Amer. med. Ass. 186, 1125—1128 (1963).

What is the Best Approach to the Primary Lesion in Breast Cancer

W. D. Rider

"In fifty cases operated upon by what we call the complete method we have been able to trace only three local recurrences." So said William S. Halsted [1] in April 1894 to the Clinical Society of Maryland. This paper opened an era of surgical tradition in the treatment of breast cancer which was to go unchallenged for half a century (Fig. 1).

THE RESULTS OF OPERATIONS FOR THE CURE OF
CANCER OF THE BREAST PERFORMED AT
THE JOHNS HOPKINS HOSPITAL
FROM JUNE, 1889, TO JANU-
ARY, 1894

BY WILLIAM S. HALSTED, M.D.,

Of Baltimore,

Professor Of Surgery In Johns Hopkins University

In fifty cases operated upon by what we call the complete method we have been able to trace only three local recurrences.

Local recurrence is a return of the disease in the field of operation, — in the apparent or buried scar. The more extensive, therefore, the operation the more liberal our interpretation of local recurrence. Until it became the custom to remove in every case the contents of the axilla, a local recurrence was understood to be a return of the cancer in the apparent scar; but now that we regularly clean out the infraclavicular and usually the supraclavicular region and remove a part, at least, of the pectoralis major muscle, a return of the disease in any part of the explored regions should be considered a local recurrence. As regionary recurrence Billroth

Fig. 1

The first major challenge came when epidemiologists [2, 3] pointed out that mortality rates were unchanged in spite of reported [4, 5, 6] steady improvement in survival rates as measured at 5 years.

Many authors [7, 8] have commented on the marked similarity of treatment results irrespective of method used, and others have shown that surgical [9, 10] skill does not influence survival rates. Finally, Phillips could show no statistically significant difference between treated and untreated breast cancer 5 year survival rates if the "count down" time was started at onset of symptoms as opposed to diagnosis and treatment.

Early diagnosis will inevitably lead to better treatment results but will this cure more patients? On the basis of mortality results it would appear that this nice logical thinking has not paid the dividends expected of it.

Why this confusion—do we ever cure breast cancer? Some authorities [12] believe that we do not, but by very conservative measures achieve highly significant long term palliation.

Much of our trouble comes from methods of selection and reliance on survival rates as the measure of our success. I would like to illustrate this aspect with the BATLEY [13] "Marbles Experiment".

A series of cloth bags were filled with beans to represent a breast.

Into each bag a predetermined number of marbles was placed, and a stage assigned according to the number of marbles. Thus 0—5 marbles represented stage I, 6—10 marbles stage II, 11—15 marbles stage III and 16—20 marbles stage IV. Each bag, representing a cancer patient, was given a finite survival depending entirely upon the numbers of marbles it contained. Two competent breast surgeons were then asked to palpate these bags and allocate them to a stage depending upon the number of marbles they felt. An average survival rate for each stage could then be calculated and the results are presented in this table:

Table

	Stage I	Stage II	Stage III	Stage IV	Overall
Doctor "A"	59	26	20	0	34
Doctor "B"	80	54	27	11	34
Predetermined	64	38	20	1	34

In the final analysis both doctors obtained exactly the same mortality rates but Doctor "B" had consistently better survival rates than Doctor "A". Had Doctor "B" practised the radical mastectomy and Doctor "A" the "lumpectomy" the deduction would be that the radical mastectomy is a far superior operation and everyone would be satisfied.

The school of conservatism in breast cancer management is growing daily since the time McWHIRTER [14] first stepped into the ring with his unprecedented simple mastectomy followed by irradiation. KAAE and JOHANSEN [15] confirmed that the McWHIRTER technique was equal to the supraradical mastectomy, CRILE [16] advocated very limited surgery and sequential management of recurrences if they develop, and MUSTAKELLIO [12] is now reporting on a larger series treated by "lumpectomy" and postoperative X-ray therapy with excellent 5 and 10 year survival rates.

Indeed, in June this year, a large international convention is being held in Strassburg on the conservative management of breast cancer. Even women's lib is getting into the scene and I have no doubt that their voice will soon be so loud that it will be impossible for a surgeon to perform the radical mastectomy in the future.

It seems to me that the radical operation and the simple procedures cure the same type of patient, and that we have not found methods of dealing with the virulent tumor. Any clinician who has had experience with breast cancer cannot fail to recognize marked differences in clinical behaviour—at one end of the scale is the old lady with a slow growing cancer that she has been hiding for years which really does not cause her death, and, at the other, the patient with the small tumour found accidentally which, by the time her primary treatment is complete has become riddled with metastases. It is tragic to have subjected the latter patient to mutilating surgery to no avail.

If there are ways and means of separating the virulent cancer from the non-virulent we have not yet made much use of it, although some clinicians have a happy knack of selecting the more benign type of cancer to operate upon and avoiding surgery in the virulent type. In this way they can achieve brilliant survival rates in their personal series [17] but unfortunately we know nothing of what happened to their "rejects".

HAAGENSEN [18], by using the triple biopsy technique for selection of operable cases, has passed his "rejects" over to RUTH GUTTMANN [19] to be treated by irradiation. In this series of "selected bad" cases she was able to show a 54% 5 year survival rate, which suggests to me that radiation is a highly effective method of therapy and maybe we should be using it more often than in the past.

In most of the so called accessible cancers radiation has proved to be of great value. I can see no inherent reason why this should not be so in another accessible cancer, at least from a radiobiological point of view, and surely, if it can be successful in the inoperable situation one would anticipate it being more effective in the "early case" where the number of malignant cells is much smaller.

For the early low grade cancer local excision alone seems to be effective particularly if it is situated in the upper outer quadrant and no nodes are palpable. This is a non-mutilating procedure suitable for the 25 year old topless go-go dancer who wants to continue her professional career. It would not be suitable for the 90 year old great grandmother who has been hiding her fungating cancer for years—she would, in all probability, be best managed by supplying her with small amounts of oestrogens, and if that failed, she could be treated by a course of radiotherapy.

Between the limits mentioned, local excision, or biopsy followed by irradiation would at least be a non-mutilating approach to the full extent of the local disease, which cannot be achieved by any other means.

The importance of sophisticated irradiation cannot be over stressed if it is to be anything more than a "cover-up" for poor surgery. The breast and its regional lymphatics comprise a difficult area to treat homogeneously due to the marked anatomical variations in size and shape. Considerable air gaps occur from place to place in this area which, if left uncorrected, give rise to large variations in absorbed dose in the regions of vital interest. If we consider the dose response curve for clinical data, derived from skin cancer treated by irradiation, it is apparent that a difference of 500 rads can cause a difference in cure rate from 50% to 85% (Fig. 2). While this data is not derived from breast cancer, there is no reason to believe that it would not apply to tumours of a skin appendage at least in general form. It is virtually impossible to achieve adequate homogeneous tumour doses likely to be effective without recourse to supervoltage irradiation as has been demonstrated by GUTTMANN [19]. Great care has to be exercised in making sure that suitable compensating filters are inserted into the beams so that the inherent errors of dose distribution are removed and homogeneous dosimetry obtained. This has certainly not been routine practice in the past, so that we can glean very little information from radiotherapy carried out at 250 K.V. other than maximum tolerated tissue doses, and some of the complications.

Finally, in connection with the radiosensitivity of breast cancer, there is much confusion due to trying to correlate the rate of disappearance with the eventual control of the cancer [20]. Some cancers respond rapidly, others very slowly—and we get no help from biopsies taken at intervals after the irradiation since "viability"

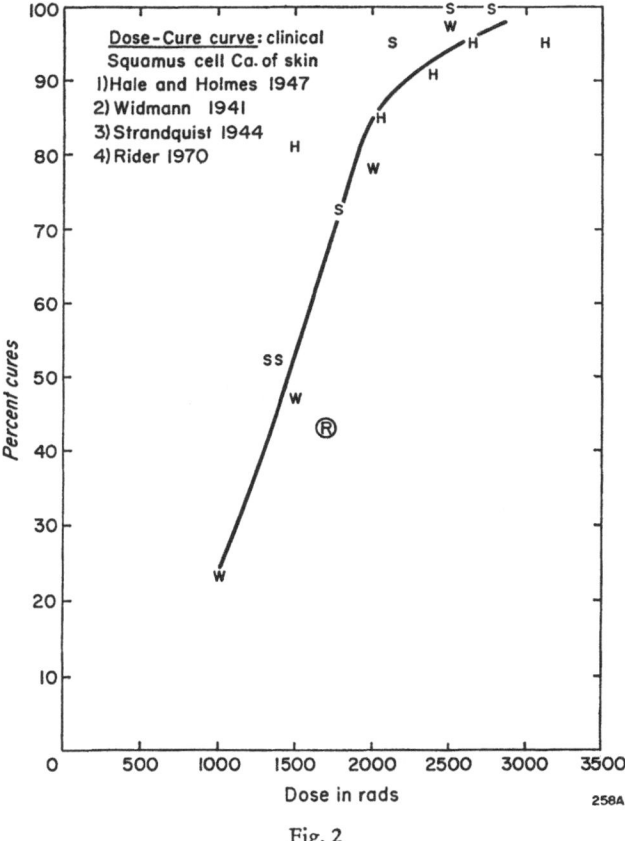

Fig. 2

cannot be assessed on histological evidence alone. This type of investigation has probably done more harm than good—the concept of tumour "sterilization" in specimens obtained surgically at some time after irradiation leading to a percentage sterilization rate. The important factor of time is ignored. Unless the tumour is allowed to complete its full cycle of regression in time, statements of sterilization are worthless. Some breast cancers can take years for complete regression, and so long as the tumour is not growing it is safe to wait and see. It follows that preoperation irradiation never makes an inoperable cancer operable.

In summary I have taken a speakers liberty of telling you my approach to the primary lesion in breast cancer. I doubt if anyone can tell you what is the right or even best method, but I believe that by more conservative methods the survival and mortality rates will be no less than in the past and women will not be mutilated. It remains for us to understand the disease better if we are ever to talk in terms of cure.

References

1. HALSTED, W. S.: The results of operation for the cure of cancer of the breast performed at the Johns Hopkins Hospital from June 1889 to January 1894. John Hopk. Hosp. Rep. 4, 297 (1894); Ann. Surg. 20, 497 (1894).
2. McKINNON, N. E.: Cancer mortality trends under different control programs. Canad. publ. Hlth J. 41, 7 (1950).
3. PARK, W. W., LEES, J. C.: The absolute curability of cancer of the breast. Surg. Gynec. Obst. 93, 129 (1951).
4. ADAIR, F. E.: Surgical problems involved in breast cancer. Moynihan Lecture. Ann. roy. Coll. Surg. Engl. 4, 360—380 (1949).
5. HARRINGTON, S. W.: Results of surgical treatment of unilateral carcinoma of breast in women. J. Amer. med. Ass. 148, 1007—1011 (1952).
6. ANGLEM, T. J., GRAY, E. B., JR.: Cancer of the breast and biological predeterminism: re-evaluation. Cancer (Philad.) 14, 1122—1126 (1961).
7. LEWISON, E. F.: Appraisal of long term results in surgical treatment of breast cancer. J. Amer. med. Ass. 186, 975—978 (1963).
8. GOLDENBERG, I. S., BAILAR, J. C. III, HAYES, M. A., LOWRY, R.: Female breast cancer: re-evaluation. Ann. Surg. 154, 397—407 (1961).
9. SMITH, S. S., MEYER, A. C.: Cancer of breast in Rockford, Illinois. Amer. J. Surg. 98, 653—656 (1959).
10. ROSAHN, P. D.: Results of treatment of carcinoma of the breast. Comparison of five year survival rates obtained by two different groups of surgeons in a community hospital. Ann. Surg. 146, 912—922 (1957).
11. PHILLIPS, A. J.: A comparison of treated and untreated cases of cancer of the breast. Brit. J. Cancer XIII, 20—25 (1959).
12. MUSTAKALLIO, S. Treatment of breast cancer by tumour extirpation and roentgen therapy instead of radical operation. J. Fac. Radiol. (Lond.) 6, 23—26 (1954) and personal communication 1972.
13. BATLEY, F.: The problem of evaluation of cancer therapy. Canad. Ass. Radiol. VI, 25—28 (1955).
14. McWHIRTER, R.: Simple mastectomy and Radiotherapy in treatment of breast cancer. Brit. J. Radiol. 28, 128 (1955).
15. KAAE, S., JOHANSEN, H.: Breast cancer: five year results; two random series of simple mastectomy with post-operative irradiation versus extended radical mastectomy. Amer. J. Roentgenol. 87, 82—88 (1962).
16. CRILE, G., JR.: Simplified treatment of cancer of breast: early results of clinical study. Ann. Surg. 153, 745—761 (1961).
17. GORDON-TAYLOR, Sir G.: Discussion. The treatment of cancer of the breast. Proc. roy. Soc. Med. 41, 118—122 (1948).
18. HAAGENSEN, C. D., COOLEY, E., KENNEDY, C. S.: Treatment of early mammary carcinoma: co-operative international study. Ann. Surg. 157, 157—161, 166—169 (1963).
19. GUTTMANN, R. J.: Survival and results after 2 million volt irradiation in treatment of primary operable carcinoma of breast with proved positive internal mammary and/or highest axillary nodes. Cancer (Philad.) 15, 383—386 (1962).
20. RIDER, W. D.: Radiosensitivity — What is it? Laryngoscope (St. Louis) LXXXI, 7, 1045—1056 (1971).

Surgical Therapy for Primary Mammary Cancer*

W. J. BURDETTE

Introduction

The disconcerting realization that carcinoma of the breast usually is disseminated when called to the attention of the clinician not only lends a sense of urgency to the solution of a major problem in oncology but also causes the physician to weigh the probable stage of the disease against the best odds offered by a variety of therapeutic regimens. Radical mastectomy has maintained a place in the forefront of best choices for therapy of localized and regional disease for over three-quarters of a century and is responsible for the first really successful management of mammary carcinoma. The remarkable advances in palliative therapy consisting of administration of hormones and ablation of endocrine glands marked a surge of hope in mid-century which so far has not been reflected in dramatically increasing the number of cures. On the other hand, the results of radiotherapy have improved with the use of megavoltage and gamma irradiation and possibly may be made even more effective by future developments of alternate choices.

The best combinations of operation and irradiation are still the subject of considerable dispute, objective response to chemotherapy is not predictable, and immunotherapy has not yet been very helpful in management.

Obviously, then, the patient presenting with possible mammary cancer cannot wait for future resolution of these uncertainties, and the best approach to the management of an individual case with primary mammary cancer must include consideration of the patient's desire to have everything done that will increase the chance of survival even at the cost of undesirable complications. This is quite a different responsibility than the selection of a regimen that gives a slightly superior result for an entire group as a whole after the extent of the disease is known. Therefore the subject of initial management of carcinoma of the breast will be approached from the standpoint of the surgeon's obligations in using the assets of operative therapy in relation to other treatment. Possible future alterations in adjuvant and operative therapy that may improve the results of contemporary therapy will also be mentioned.

The assumption will be made throughout the discussion that all therapy is based on biopsy findings, complete ablation of a neoplasm is curative, radiotherapy can eradicate mammary cancer in lymph nodes if the volume is not too great, therapy adjuvant to operation is likely to be more effective when the number of neoplastic

* Aided by grant CA 05831 from the Public Health Service, U. S. Department of Health, Education and Welfare.

cells remaining is smaller, and curative and cosmetic operations are not necessarily mutually exclusive.

Localized and regional disease are responsive both to surgical and irradiation therapy, but cure of disseminated disease awaits the successful application of additional modes of therapy. When mammary cancer first comes to the attention of the clinician, the disease is localized in approximately one-quarter of the cases, about one-sixth of the patients have regional nodes invaded with cancer, and two-thirds of the patients have metastases beyond the axilla. At least two-thirds of those patients

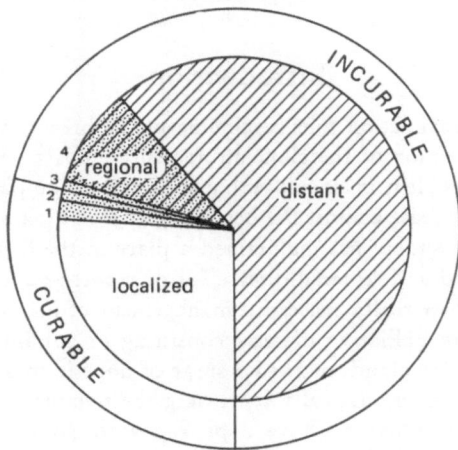

Fig. 1. Diagram showing the extent of mammary carcinoma when first seen by the physician. No specific percentages have been assigned, since this varies from one study to the next within broad limits. However, these general relationships hold for most data collected within the recent past. Localized and regional disease without distant metastases are the only two classes of lesions that are currently amenable to cure by operation and/or irradiation. A portion of the regional (1, 2, 3, 4) disease may be eradicated by surgical therapy (1), and there is suggestive evidence that postoperative irradiation will give some additional cures (2). However, regional disease is at times refractory to both ablative therapy and irradiation (3). When distant metastases are present as well, cures are rarely obtained (4). It is unlikely that any combinations of irradiation therapy and surgery will extend the number of cures very much as long as the present situation exists. For any appreciable improvement in current results to ensue, it is obvious from the diagram that one must find means (a) for diagnosing the disease early in order to shift the temporal frame and thus bring cases to the attention of the surgeon and radiologist for therapy, when they are localized or (b) for treating patients with distant metastases successfully

with regional disease also have disseminated disease, and not even all patients who are treated with only regional disease survive. There is suggestive evidence (sometimes contested [17]) that the addition of radiotherapy will salvage a small number of patients with regional disease who would not be cured by operation alone [18, 50].

Most discussion in recent decades has centered on the relative value of operative and irradiation therapy alone and combined. The accompanying diagram (Fig. 1) suggests that a solution satisfactory to all therapists about the proper roles of each will result in very little change in the number of cures. Short of prevention, it will be

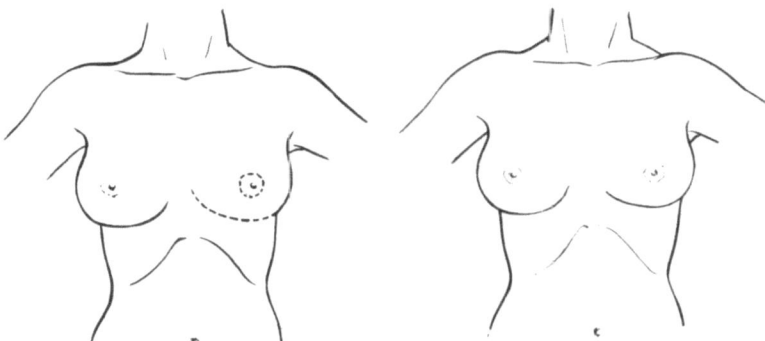

Fig. 2. Subcutaneous mastectomy with insertion of a prosthesis for augmentation is a possible method for treating precancers and localized cancers of the breast. When necessary, the nipple can be transplanted, and bilateral procedures offer no additional problems. Both axillary and inferior extensions of the glandular tissue are removed

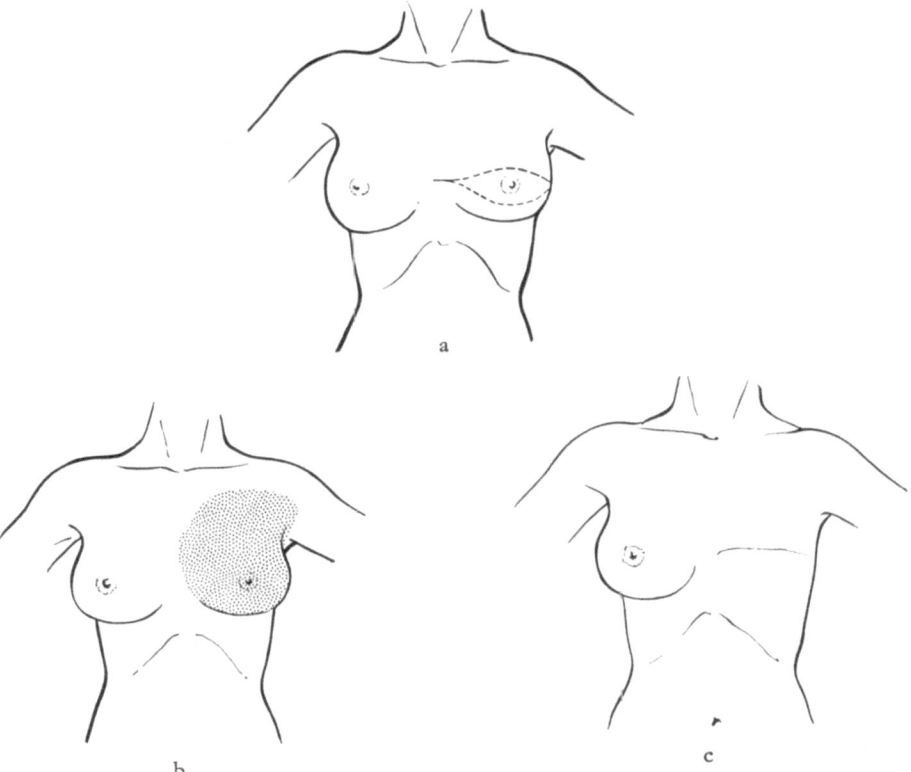

Fig. 3. Simple mastectomy, which sometimes is referred to as total mastectomy to emphasize the necessity for excising the entire breast, has been done for many years for localized and precancerous lesions and may be combined with irradiation for cancer when regional spread is suspected. After incising the skin (A), it is reflected for considerable distance (B) in order to accomplish adequate removal of all mammary tissue. A generous wedge of skin is excised with the nipple, but muscles and axillary contents are preserved, leaving a relatively small scar (C)

necessary to add successful treatment of disseminated cancer or to shift the temporal frame so that the numbers of localized lesions coming to the attention of the surgeon are greatly increased by improved diagnostic measures. The latter will be valueless unless curative treatment for early manifestations of localized cancer or precancer is given immediately. Safe cosmetic repair with augmentation undoubtedly would make ablative therapy more acceptable both to the physician and his patient.

Operative Approaches

In addition to biopsy, necessary in every case for diagnosis, the surgical procedures available are fairly well standardized and not great in number. Local excision of a neoplasm, sometimes referred to by the inelegant term, lumpectomy, has the descriptive disadvantage that the extent of resection is not defined and also is a procedure whose value is questioned by many even when combined with irradiation

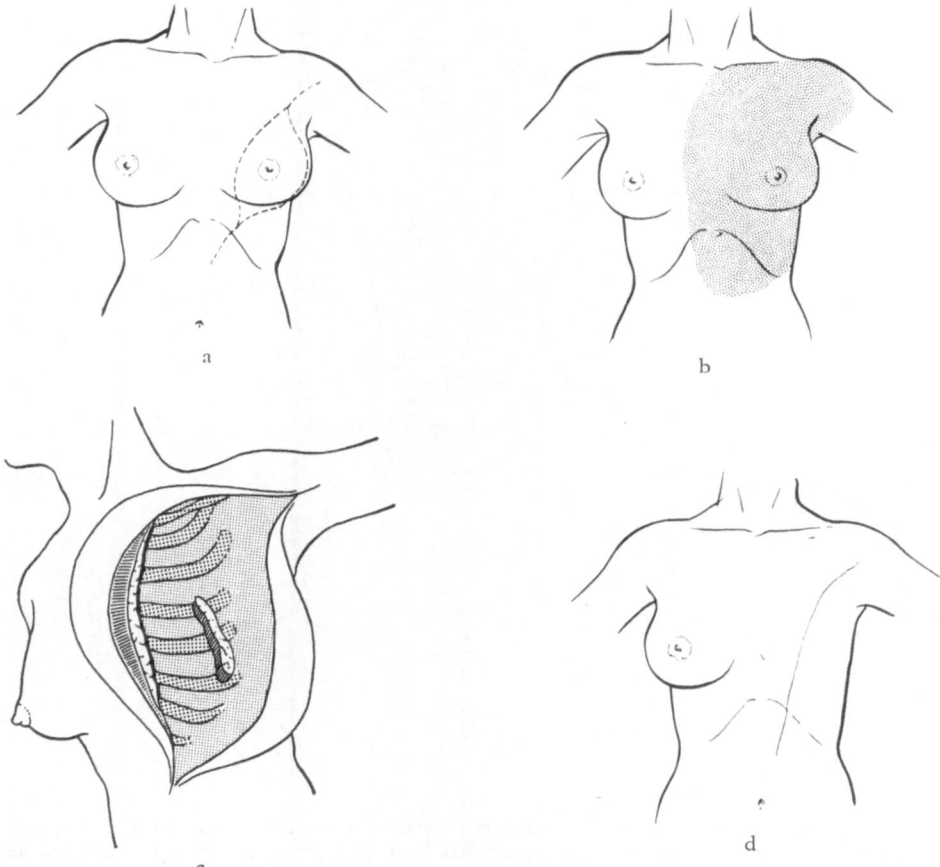

Fig. 4. Radical mastectomy consists of removing the breast, excising a generous amount of skin (A), developing flaps covering a wide area (B), and resection of pectoralis major and minor (C), the deep fascia including anterior rectus sheath, and the axillary contents

therapy. Subcutaneous mastectomy with plastic augmentation for precancerous lesions or non-invasive carcinoma is looked upon with more favor now than in the past as a possible means for treatment, although adequacy of the procedure has not been proved (Fig. 2). Simple mastectomy (sometimes called total mastectomy) consists of removal of all mammary tissue and excision of nipple and ellipse of skin with preservation of pectoralis major and minor and without axillary dissection (Fig. 3). The classical radical mastectomy (Fig. 4) includes removal of the entire breast, nipple, and surrounding skin with extensive undermining of flaps; removal of fascia including the superior portion of anterior rectus sheath; extirpation of pectoralis major and minor muscles; and resection of axillary contents. The modified radical mastectomy (Fig. 5)

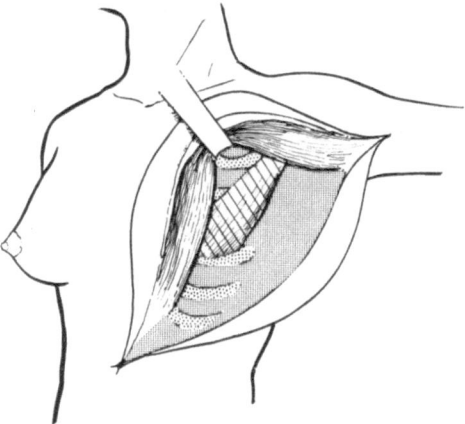

Fig. 5. The modified radical mastectomy preserves the pectoralis major and minor or the pectoralis major. Extended radical mastectomy includes removal of internal mammary nodes and/or supraclavicular nodes. Note the extensive undermining of skin and the extent of the operation. A skin graft may be necessary in order to close a defect brought about to prevent local recurrence. Removal of pectoralis minor is advocated in order to remove interpectoral nodes more adequately

consists of total mastectomy, removal of axillary contents, and preservation of one or both pectoral muscles. Any description of this operation should include information about whether pectoralis major or pectoralis major and minor are left in place. The extended radical mastectomy adds resection of internal mammary nodes and/or extension of resection of nodes to those above the clavicle. The super-radical operation, no longer performed, included extensive dissection in mediastinum and neck. Resection of solitary metastatic lesions in the lung is a procedure applicable only to the unusual case.

The most successful therapy other than operation is the use of megavoltage and gamma irradiation (that have supplanted kilovoltage). It is usually given through one to four ports (Fig. 6): mammary, internal mammary, supraclavicular and highest portion of axilla, and posterior. Oophorectomy or irradiation of the ovaries in pre- and/or postmenopausal women have been used as an adjunct to operation, and chemotherapy and immunotherapy continue to attract attention as possible adjuvants to ablative therapy. Even if the multiplicity of possible quantitative doses of drugs alone and in combination; quality and dosage schedules of irradiation; and methodologies for possible immunotherapy are omitted, there remain at least 1568 possible ways for treating carcinoma of the breast (Table 1). This explains in part why it has been rather difficult to focus on the best regimen for treating the disease when clinically localized in breast and regional nodes.

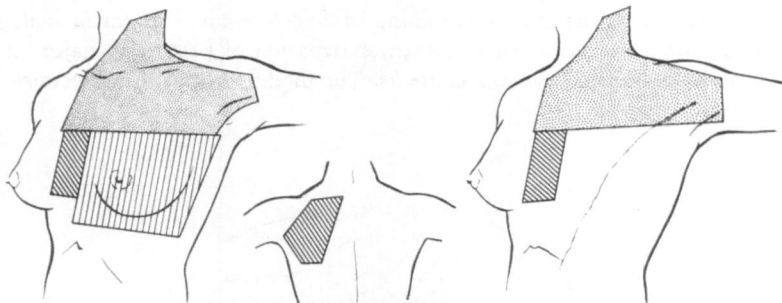

Fig. 6. Fields used for irradiating patients with mammary carcinoma. Preoperative irradiation may be given through ports illustrated on the left and postoperative therapy through those on the right. The posterior field may be added at times

Table 1. Combinations of therapy for mammary carcinoma

Ablation	Radiation		Adjuvant therapy	
	Type	Sequence		
None	None	Preoperative	None	None
Local excision	Breast	Postoperative	Chemo-therapy	Immuno-therapy
Subcutaneous mastectomy	Lymphatics			
Simple mastectomy	Axillary			
Radical mastectomy	Internal mammary			
Modified radical mastectomy	Supraclavicular			
Extended radical mastectomy				

Therapy Adjuvant to Operation

NISSEN-MEYER et al. [44] as well as others, have been optimistic in their advocacy of irradiation of the ovaries as a useful adjunct to ablative and/or irradiation therapy. However, other objective clinical trials carried out as prospective studies, such as those of RAVDIN et al. [49] failed to substantiate the value of oöphorectomy as a useful adjuvant to radical mastectomy (Table 2). The prospective clinical trials to assess the value of specific types of chemotherapy carried out in the United States by FISHER et al. [13, 14, 15, 16, 17] (Tables 2, 3, and 4) yielded only the suggestion that TSPA may be useful in treating patients with more than three nodes involved in the axilla when radical mastectomy is carried out as a primary form of treatment. Since oöphorectomy in the premenopausal patient and chemotherapy both have undesirable

Table 2. Survival five years after radical mastectomy [a]

Nodes	Operation and oöphorectomy		Operation and TSPA		Operation alone	
	Number of patients	% Survival	Number of patients	% Survival	Number of patients	% Survival
Negative	30	77	22	68	17	77
Positive	44	39	26	46	20	40
1—3+	18	61	11	64	5	60
4+	26	23	15	33	15	33
Total	74	54	48	56	37	57

[a] RAVDIN, LEWISON, SLACK, DAO, GARDNER, STATE, FISHER, et al. [49].

Table 3. Results of chemotherapy adjuvant to radical mastectomy

Group	Survival (5 years)			
	TSPA		Control	
	No.	%	No.	%
Premenopausal				
nodes —	55	80	54	81
1—3 nodes +	21	65	24	67
≥4 nodes +	23	57 [a]	37	24
Postmenopausal				
nodes —	151	74	165	76
1—3 nodes +	88	61	66	61
≥3 nodes +	76	37	60	32

[a] $P < 0.05$
FISHER, RAVDIN, AUSMAN, SLACK, MOORE, NOER, et al. [17].

Table 4. Results of chemotherapy adjuvant to radical mastectomy [a]

Group	Recurrence (36 months)					
	TSPA		5 FU		Control	
	No.	%	No.	%	No.	%
Premenopausal						
negative nodes	57	16	42	14	23	17
positive nodes	88	61	49	61	28	61
Postmenopausal						
negative nodes	193	12	135	14	38	16
positive nodes	175	50	111	55	62	50

[a] FISHER, RAVDIN, AUSMAN, SLACK, MOORE, NOER et al. [15].

consequences and neither is known to cure the disease at the present time, the wisdom
of using them routinely as part of the primary treatment of cancer thought to be confined to breast and/or regional nodes is open to question.

Problems in utilizing kinetic parameters for designing and carrying out chemotherapy related to variations in these measurements from one neoplasm to the next
[42] and the absence of suitable drugs specific for mammary cancer tempers any
enthusiasm for the use of drugs along with operation for cancer of the breast. However, success in the treatment of other types of neoplastic diseases with adjuvant
chemotherapy such as Wilm's tumors and rhabdomyosarcomas suggests that chemotherapy may ultimately prove to be a very useful form of adjunctive management. It
is generally agreed [34, 42] that both chemotherapy and immunotherapy should be
most effective when the number of neoplastic cells is smallest. Therefore operation
should yield the most optimum conditions for adjuvant therapy to be successful by
reducing the number of cancer cells to a minimum. Of course, to be weighed against
the possible desirable effects of chemotherapy is the possible damage to immunologic
mechanisms preventing dissemination at the time of operative manipulation.

The reports of tumor-associated antigens, homologous RNA both in polysome
fractions of human mammary cancer and murine mammary-tumor virus, and visu-
alization of candidate viruses in human milk and mammary tissue [12, 34, 52], tempt
speculation that proper manipulation of tumor-associated antigens and both cellular
and humoral defenses against them will provide useful methods for diagnosing and
treating mammary cancer [34, 52]. However, many problems are involved in utilizing both immunotherapy and chemotherapy at present. The responses of mammary
tumors in binding and responding to hormones reported by JENSEN [37] suggest that
molecular maneuvers may ultimately provide useful information for prognosticating
response of mammary neoplasms to other forms of therapy in addition to hormones,
but these approaches have not yet matured.

From these considerations it is apparent that the contemporary therapist must
turn to the best combination of operation and radiotherapy and all that diagnostic
measures such as xerography, thermography, mammography, and ultrasound have to
offer [10, 11] to provide the best chance for cure. Currently these latter techniques
and micromorphologic criteria offer the only practical way to move in the direction
of increasing the proportion of localized neoplasms found at the time of diagnosis in
comparison to those disseminated. As progress in estimating risks more precisely is

Table 5. Effect of radiotherapy after radical mastectomy on survival for 5 years [a]

Status	Postoperative radiotherapy		Adjuvant TSPA		Control	
	No.	%	No.	%	No.	%
Premenopausal	30	55	42	64	34	62
Postmenopausal	165	56	78	60	79	62
Negative nodes	50	74	28	79	33	82
Positive nodes	115	49	50	33	46	48

[a] FISHER, SLACK, CAVANAUGH, GARDNER, RAVDIN et al. [17].

made, this may enhance the value of radiohistodiagnosis by helping to indicate those patients who should have definitive treatment for early cancer or precancer [61].

Radiotherapy in conjunction with radical mastectomy has been reported to improve the results of this procedure [18, 50]. However, a comparative prospective study [49] carried out in the United States failed to reveal additional benefit from irradiation after the radical procedure (Table 5). Nevertheless, it would seem prudent to include post-operative irradiation when there is considerable likelihood that regional nodes are involved.

Selection of Operative Management

After it was advocated by MOORE, GROSS, BANKS, and FOLKMAN, KÜSTER carried out a systematic axillary dissection in the treatment of all cases of cancer of the breast, and HEIDENHAIN removed the superficial portion of the pectoral muscles and at times the pectoralis minor muscles [13]. Unfortunately local recurrence after operation for mammary carcinoma persisted as a feature in as many as four out of five cases. Using radical mastectomy, HALSTED was able to report approximately a ten-fold improvement in local recurrence, although improvement in cures was not dramatic [26, 27, 28, 29].

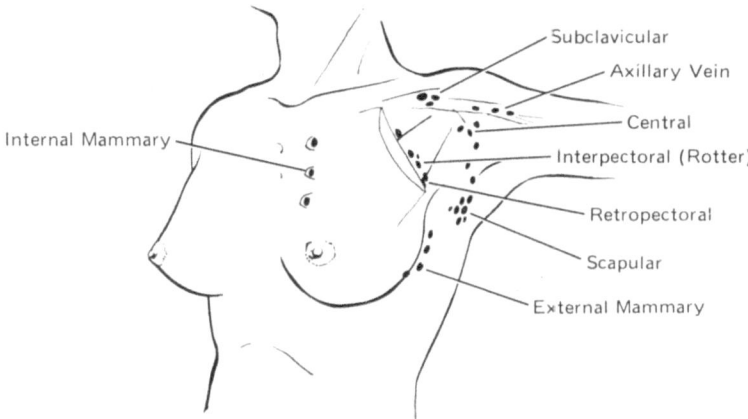

Fig. 7. Simplified diagram showing distribution of regional nodes

The basis for the radical operation was the supposed orderly progression of spread through the lymphatics and the relative unimportance of hematogenous dissemination (Fig. 7). The illustrations (Fig. 8) and data (Fig. 9) published by HALSTED clearly reflect that he advocated wide excision of skin and neoplasm with regional lymphatics in order to prevent local recurrence and to circumscribe the neoplasm and its peripheral extensions (Fig. 10). Based on the work of others, the rationale of HALSTED proved not to be entirely correct. A pragmatic approach to therapy rather than adherence to authoritarian concepts now seems to be preferable. However, this implies the disagreeable task of choosing between uncertain alternatives. Most of the problem lies in having to balance undesirable sequelae against increasing the chance of survival by proper management of regional nodes. Possible means for prognostica-

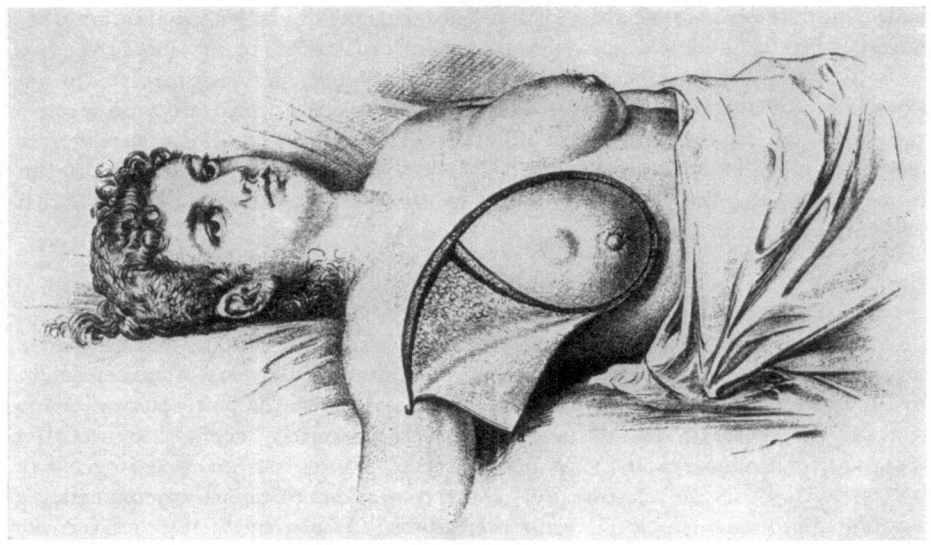

a

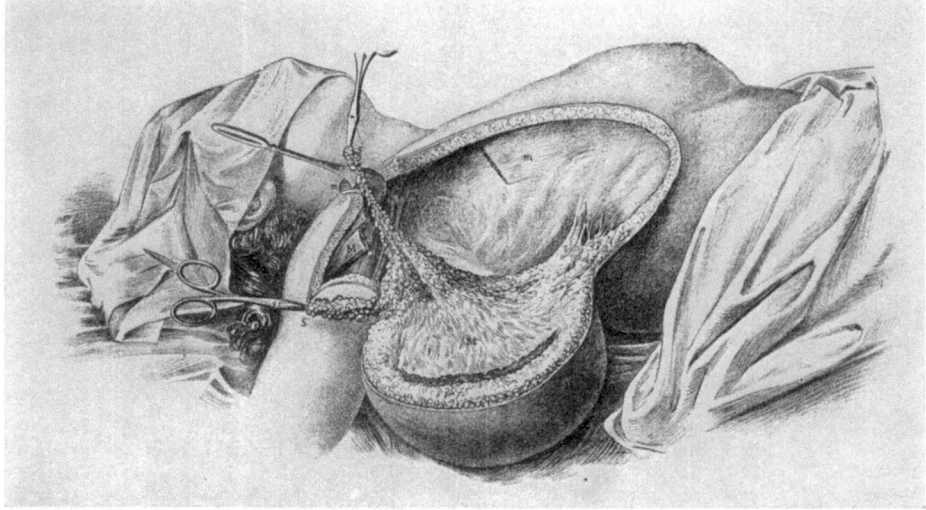

b

Fig. 8. Reproductions from original illustrations used by Halsted showing wide excision of skin (A) to prevent local recurrence and the radical nature of the mastectomy (B) which he practiced. (By permission of the original publishers)

tion on the basis of clinical findings are the size of the primary tumor [16] and its location [30], the presence of nodes on physical examination [21], and whether axillary nodes are positive for tumor when examined microscopically at the time of axillary dissection [2, 21, 30].

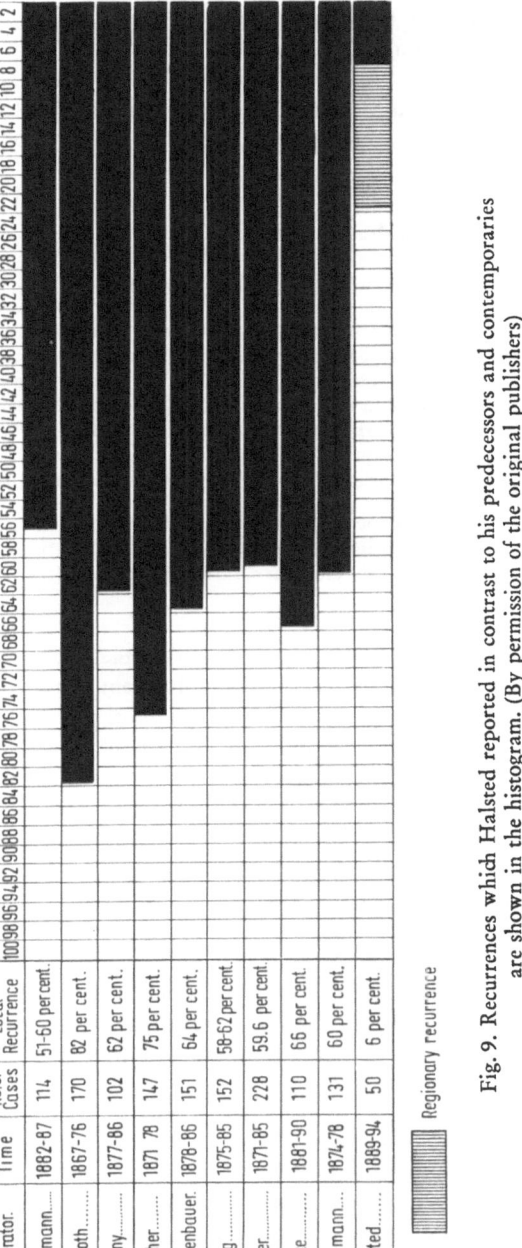

Fig. 9. Recurrences which Halsted reported in contrast to his predecessors and contemporaries are shown in the histogram. (By permission of the original publishers)

The size of the primary lesion [16] can vary within broad limits without prognostic significance. The work of HANDLEY [30] at the Middlesex Hospital in London provides an anatomical basis for the relationship between site of primary carcinoma and regional spread (Table 6). Clearly the location of the lesion has prognostic implications because medial and central lesions carry a very high risk of mediastinal involvement. When axillary nodes are invaded with metastatic disease, the chance that supraclavicular nodes and/or mammary nodes are also involved too, is increased considerably.

THE OPERATION

Though the area of disease extend from cranium to knee, breast cancer in the broad sense is a local affection, and there comes to the surgeon an encouragement to greater endeavor with the cognition that the metastases to bone, to pleura, to liver are probably parts of the whole, and that the involvements are almost invariably by process of lymphatic permeation, and not embolic by way of the blood. If extension, the most rapid, takes place beneath the skin along the fascial planes, we must remove not only a very large amount of skin and a much larger area of subcutaneous fat and fascia, but also strip the sheaths from the upper part of the rectus, the ser-ratus magnus, the subscapularis, and, at times, from parts of the latissimus dorsi and the teres major. Both pectoral muscles are, of course, removed.

Fig. 10. The text in Halsted's papers clearly indicated that his rationale for radical mast-ectomy depended on the assumption that carcinoma of the breast spreads almost entirely through lymphatic channels and very rarely by way of the blood stream

Although a surprising number of cases have palpable nodes without any of them containing metastatic cancer, clinical nodal involvement should lead to serious con-sideration of ablation of axillary contents for diagnosis of external disease and therapy. Since nodes may contain tumor when they are not palpable clinically, this circumstance combined with the uncertainty about whether management after nodes become pal-pable is superior to prophylactic management leads to the viewpoint that the axilla should be explored in all cases [21]. However, such a decision carries with it the risk of additional complications of therapy such as edema of the arm and limitation of motion. Studies such as those of BRUCE [4] and HEALEY [33] (Tables 7 and 8) suggest that both irradiation and operative therapy lead to these two complications. When axillary operation is carried out without irradiation, edema is more frequent com-plication than when irradiation is carried out alone whereas the reverse is true for limitation of motion. On the other hand, irradiation carries very little risk of in-creasing the number of patients with edema when it follows extirpation of axillary contents.

When the merits of various ablative procedures are reviewed, it soon becomes apparent that appropriate selection of survival figures reported by various authors [5, 7, 24, 31, 38, 39, 59] can be used to support any therapeutic regimen of operation with or without radiotherapy provided preselection of patients is not required and protocols for management are not followed invariably in judging their validity (Table 9). In the past, attempts to improve the results of radical mastectomy gravitated in opposite directions. WANGENSTEEN et al. [56] attempted to extend the operation to supraclavicular and internal mammary nodes. On the other hand, HAAGENSEN, STOUT, et al. [24, 25] restricted the indications for operation in a con-servative direction. Quite clearly, the latter has been more successful, and the super-radical approach has been abandoned by most surgeons [6, 55], although mediastinal

Table 6. Invasion of lymph nodes by mammary carcinoma

Location of primary	All patients %		Patients with axillary nodes [a] %	
	No. of patients	Internal mammary nodes involved	No. of patients	Internal mammary nodes involved
Inner	158	31	67	51
Central	90	47	64	59
Outer	252	19	155	28
Total	500		286	

[a] HANDLEY [30]

Table 7. Late complications in 395 patients [a]

Procedure	%	
	Edema of arm	Limitation of shoulder motion
Simple mastectomy and irradiation	5	14
Radical mastectomy alone	10	4

[a] BRUCE [4]

Table 8. Lymphedema complicating management of mammary carcinoma [a]

Therapy	No. of patients	% With edema > 15%
Operation	37	40.5
Preop. radiation and operation	57	41.4
Operation and postop. radiation	134	41.1
Radiation	40	17.5
Other	3	100.0

[a] HEALEY [33]

exploration has not been entirely forsaken under special circumstances by URBAN et al. [54]. As time has progressed, the clinical criteria of HAAGENSEN and STOUT [25] (Table 10) for inoperable lesions and the custom of considering as operable only those in the Columbia Clinical Classification A and B have been widely accepted indications for radical or modified radical mastectomy.

When a diagnosis of mammary carcinoma is made from radiographic studies and physical examination, biopsy of the breast should be carried out in the operating room where additional operative therapy is possible immediately. Removal of the entire neoplasm is obviously desirable, and this is most likely to be accomplished when mastectomy is performed. The addition of axillary dissection yields additional

Table 9. Five-year survival for mammary cancer after different methods of therapy [a]

Author	KENNEDY and MILLER [39]		KAAE and JOHANSEN [23, 38]		WILLIAMS and CURWEN [23, 59]		HANDLEY and THACHEREY [23, 31]		BUTCHER [5, 23]		HAAGENSEN and COOLEY [23]		DAHL-IVERSON and TOBIASEEN [7, 23]	
Procedure	Simple mastectomy minimal irradiation		Total mastectomy radiation		Modified mastectomy radiation postoperative		Modified mastectomy [b]		Radical mastectomy [b]		Radical mastectomy [b]		Extended radical mastectomy [b]	
	No.	%	No.	%	No.	%	No.	%	No.	%	No.	%	No.	%
Stage A	115	62	159	70	68	72	77	75	164	76	344	84	277	77
Stage B	34	41	28	50	57	60	58	57	65	48	138	59	61	48
Total cases	212	45	199	64	142	63	143	65	225	60	556	72	366	70

[a] Modified from HAAGENSEN et al. [23].
[b] Some with irradiation.

information about involvement of axillary nodes with the added advantage of extirpation of metastatic disease in this location when present. Complications such as limited motion and edema are not only confined to the surgical approach to the axilla but also occur in some cases treated with irradiation, as has been mentioned. Modification of the radical mastectomy by leaving pectoralis major, and possibly pectoralis minor, muscles intact deserves some consideration in view of the reports of PATEY and DYSON [45], HANDLEY [31], MADDEN [40], et al. The preservation of pectoralis major seems a reasonable compromise, since adequate dissection of the axillary contents still can be carried out. The likelihood either of overlooking involved regional nodes or impairment of motion in the shoulder does not seem to be great. On the other hand, examination of data such as those presented by HAAGENSEN (Table 11)

Table 10. Columbia clinical classification

Stage	A	B	C (One or more)
Primary neoplasm	+	+	Fixed
Axillary nodes	—	< 2.5 Cm.	≥ 2.5 Cm.; fixed
Skin	—	—	Ulceration; limited edema (< 1/3)

Table 11. Relative number of axillary nodes

Group of nodes	Number of cases with nodes	Total number of nodes	Mean number of nodes	% cases with involved nodes
Central	182	2199	12.1	39.6
Interpectoral	97	262	1.4	17.5
Axillary vein	179	1948	10.7	15.1
Scapular	152	1061	5.8	9.9
Subclavicular	169	641	3.5	8.9
External mammary	96	311	1.7	6.2

HAAGENSEN [21]

shows that the interpectoral group of nodes is involved with cancer much more often than would be anticipated on the basis of the number of nodes usually present in this location. Because of this, it seems advisable to remove the pectoralis minor in order to deal more effectively with the interpectoral nodes.

The compromise of performing simple mastectomy and treating axillary nodes with postoperative irradiation has been the subject of many reports since the original report of McWHIRTER [41] from the Royal Infirmary in Edinburgh. WILLIAMS et al. [59], DEN BESTEN and ZIFFREN [8], DEVITT and BEATTIE [9] and KAAE and JOHANSEN [38] are among those who feel that these studies fail to indicate superiority of simple mastectomy and postoperative irradiation over radical mastectomy. Others take the opposite view [21, 22, 23, 51, 56]. MUSTAKALLIO [43], PORRITT [48], PETERS [46], HOERR [35], ACKERMAN et al. [1], and some have suggested that local excision of the neoplasm followed by irradiation will cure as many patients as more radical surgery.

In choosing among the more conservative alternatives to the type of radical mastectomy practiced by MEYER and HALSTED, the compromise of modified radical mastectomy seems a reasonable one as long as pectoralis minor muscle is removed and the criteria for inoperability proposed by HAAGENSEN *et al.* are followed. The reduced rate of complications and improved appearance after the modified procedure compared to radical mastectomy in part offset the objections to this more conservative operative approach. Possibly the chief objection to radical mastectomy is that an axillary dissection is carried out in some patients who do not have involvement of regional nodes. In that case, irradiation postoperatively is not advocated when modified radical mastectomy is performed and no axillary nodes are found to contain neoplastic cells, whereas it is mandatory after simple mastectomy or local excision plus irradiation. Simple mastectomy and irradiation are followed by serious com-

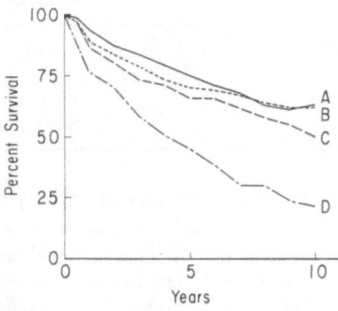

Fig. 11. In 10 years results [18] of preoperative irradiation and radical mastectomy in 419 patients with disturbed breasts (B) show survival figures about the same as those in 246 patients without previous surgical management treated primarily with radical mastectomy (A). Axillary nodes were invaded in 29% of the former group and 9% of the latter. The lower survival figures for radical mastectomy and postoperatvive irradiation (C) and simple mastectomy and postoperative irradiation (D) are understandable in this series [18, 58], since postoperative irradiation was carried out in 353 cases with positive axillary nodes in 63% of the cases and simple mastectomy as an aid to the radiologist in treating 138 cases of advanced (grade III) disease

plications at times [1]. For these reasons and because of the greater experience with radical mastectomy, it is believed that the primary procedure for carcinoma of the breast should be modified radical mastectomy.

In view of the experience with extended operative therapy by CACERES [6], VERONESI [55], DAHL-IVERSEN [7], *et al.*, the evidence does not seem compelling that operation should be extended either to supraclavicular or internal mammary nodes. However, increased frequency of involvement of internal mammary nodes in central and medial lesions and when axillary nodes are involved [21, 30], suggests that irradiation should be carried out postoperatively when the primary cancer is located centrally or medially. The same increased frequency of involvement of supraclavicular nodes when axillary nodes contain cancer suggests that postoperative irradiation not only should be carried out through internal mammary port but also through supraclavicular high axillary port (with addition of a posterior port when necessary) if axillary nodes contain neoplastic cells.

Preoperative irradiation may have a place in therapy when the breast has been disturbed by biopsy, trauma, or infection. WHITE and FLETCHER [18, 58] have reported that the number of local recurrences and overall results were much improved by preoperative irradiation in these patients. The results with and without pre-operative irradiation over a period of 10 years (Fig. 11) are not comparable, how-ever, because patients receiving preoperative irradiation had axillary nodes involved in greater numbers.

In patients with advanced disease, irradiation therapy may be very helpful, and the surgeon can offer useful adjunctive therapy to this irradiation by removing the entire breast or local recurrences when this facilitates the course of irradiation. In addition, the surgeon may occasionally encounter a patient with solitary pulmonary metastasis with primary lesion controlled and no other manifestations of the disease who can be cured by resection of the pulmonary lesion.

Management of Precancer and Carcinoma *in Situ*

The combination of mammography and/or xerography along with whole-organ section [20] makes it apparent that many neoplasms are multiple [53]. This has focused attention on certain lesions such as noninvasive intraductal carcinoma which are not always considered malignant or called by that name when seen by all pathol-ogists (Fig. 12). Lobular carcinoma carries a high risk of multiple neoplasms and bilateral involvement [36]. Success in diagnosing neoplastic lesions early in their course has improved with the advent of mammography and xerography, and the augmentation operation [19] offers the possibility of a plastic procedure that restores the appearance of the breast when a localized cancer or precancerous lesion is re-moved. In addition, a number of conditions are known to carry a high risk [47, 60, 61] for mammary carcinoma. For example increased risk is associated with spinster-hood, earlier menarche, older age, postmenopausal state, fewer pregnancies, late age at first pregnancy, shorter breast feeding, and oöphorectomy; and mammary car-cinoma is also associated with antecedent contralateral carcinoma, racial derivation (e. g.; Caucasian), and the *A*, *ss*, and wet ear-wax genes. The importance of family history in relation to risk is indicated by data from the M. D. Anderson Hospital given in Tables 12 and 13. When these risks are combined with the presence of presumptive evidence from xerograms (Fig. 13) and the diagnosis of carcinoma *in situ* or a precancer, serious consideration must be given to combined ablative and plastic operation. (Although originating in a different context, Halsted's statement, "I should not care to say, 'Beware of the man with the plastic operation'" may be equally applicable to the minimal lesion.) This approach should be carried out as a careful prospective clinical trial and not as a current fashion for isolated cases. Caution is suggested by complications such as distortion from circular fibrosis, infections, and sloughs of the skin that occur after subcutaneous mastectomy and repair. It is not known whether one can increase the numbers of cures sufficiently to offset any possible risk limited as it is by preservation of the nipple. Since reports by FREEMAN [19] and others justify some degree of optimism about cosmetic results, possibilities

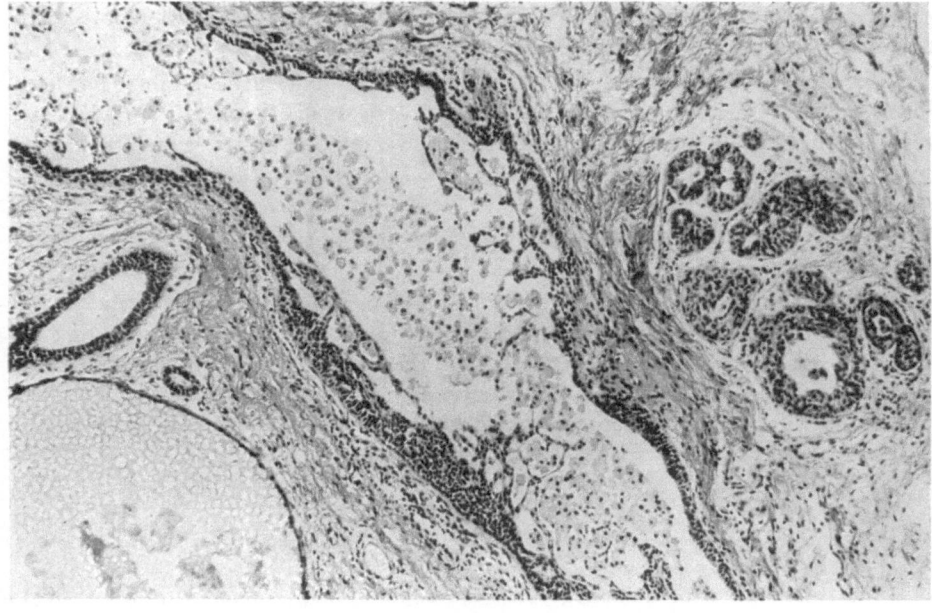

a

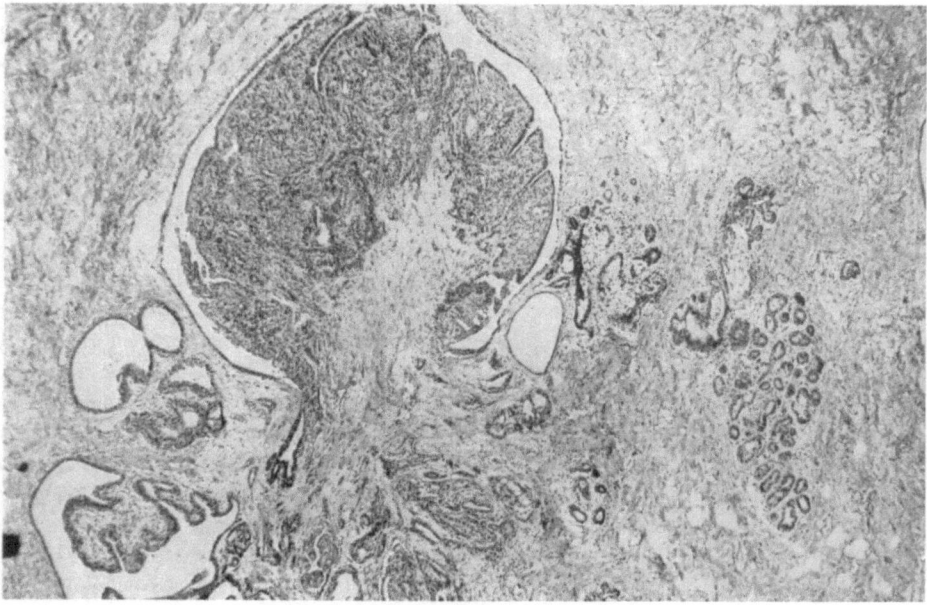

b

Fig. 12. Type of microscopic picture seen in many breasts which are thought to contain localized cancer or precancer. In these sections from a single breast, cyst (A), sclerosing adenosis (B), fibroadenoma (C), and configuration called intraductal carcinoma without invasion (D) by some pathologists are seen

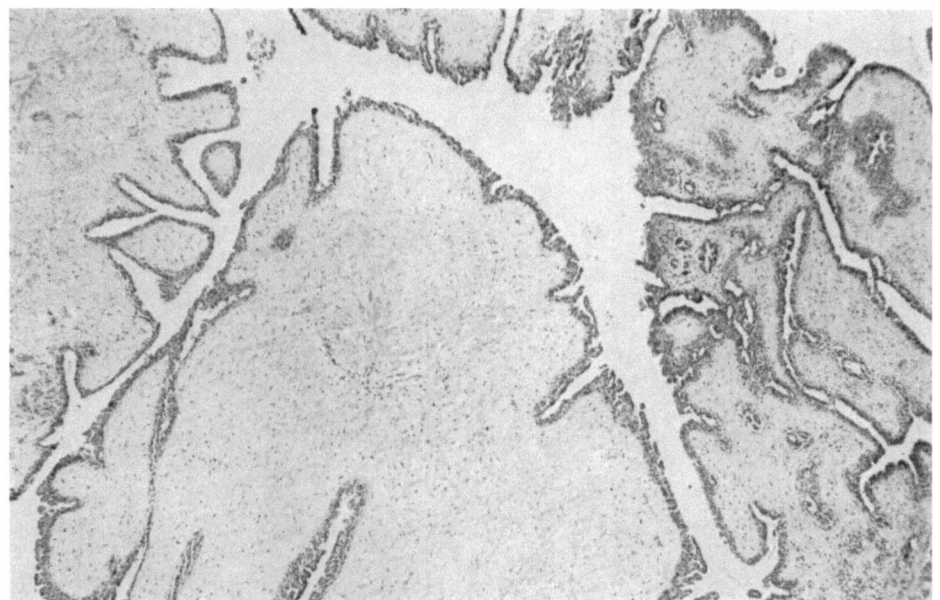

c

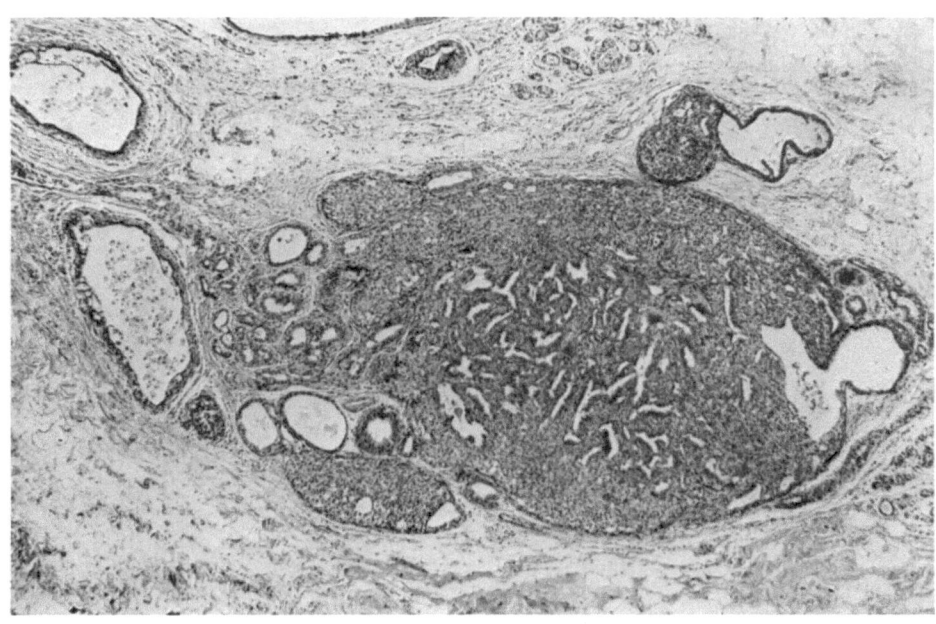

d

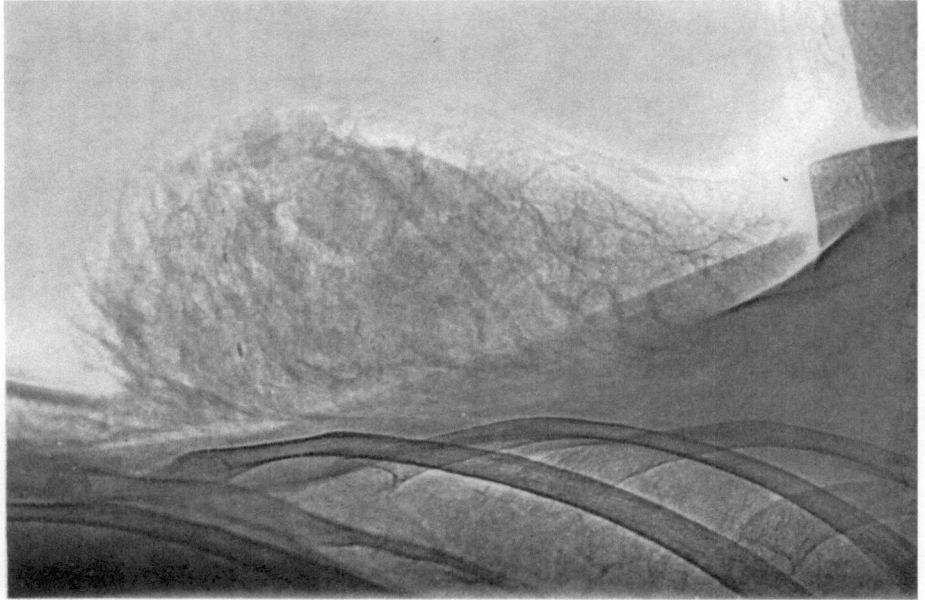

a

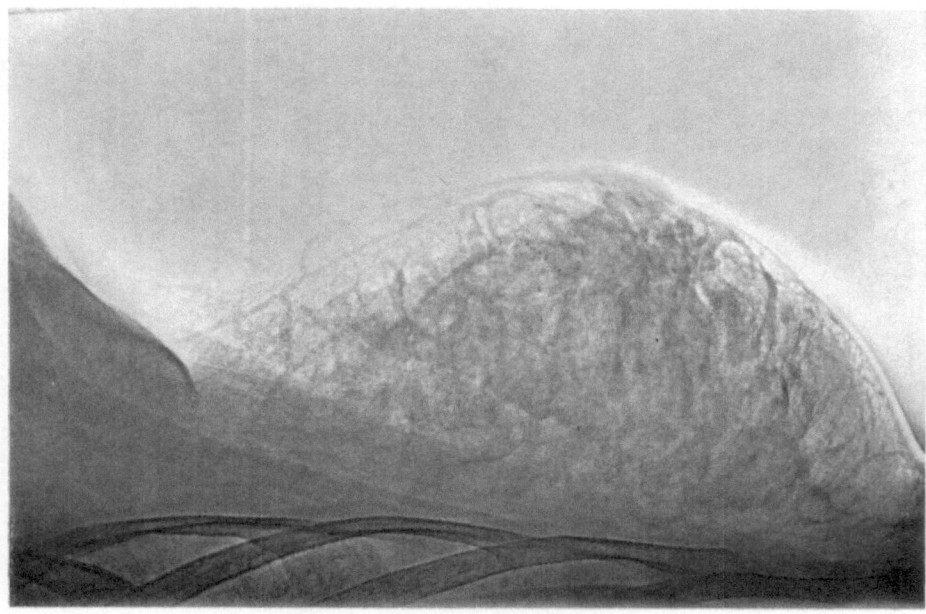

b

Fig. 13. Xerograms showing fibroadenoma in the left breast (A) and fine calcifications distributed throughout both breasts (A and B). Microscopic sections illustrated in Fig. 12 are from the same patient. This patient was treated by bilateral subcutaneous mastectomy with augmentation. Similar microscopic findings were present in both breasts

Table 12. History of cancer in relatives of patients with cancer

Relation to proband	Breast (6812) %	Colon and rectum (2831) %	Lung (3560) %
Father	8.1	7.2	7.7
Mother	9.8	9.6	8.5
Sibling	13.5	16.5	15.5
Other	13.9	9.8	6.2
Positive	0.5	0.9	0.4
Total positive	45.7	44.0	38.3

Table 13. History of cancer of the same type in relatives of patients with cancer

Relation to proband	Breast (4839) %	Colon and rectum (1888) %	Lung (2519) %
Father	0.1	1.5	1.0
Mother	4.0	2.0	0.5
Sibling	5.0	2.8	3.8
Other	5.1	1.7	0.9
Positive	0.2	0.7	0.3
Total positive	14.3	8.6	6.4

of the procedure for managing potentially neoplastic and localized lesions deserve careful trial.

Possible indications for subcutaneous mastectomy with replacement are prior proved malignancy in one breast and suspicious mammogram in the remaining breast; progressive nodularity in patients with a two or three-fold increased empiric risk; lobular carcinoma *in situ;* noninvasive intraductal carcinoma; and cystosarcoma phylloides. Possibility of multicentric origin and advantages of symmetry when two prostheses are in place make bilateral operation, particularly in lobular carcinoma, a matter for careful consideration whenever subcutaneous mastectomy is planned.

Conclusions

1. A respectable percentage of additional cures of mammary cancer will depend on increased diagnostic accuracy earlier in the course of the disease and willingness to extirpate early lesions along with the development of effective endocrine therapy, chemotherapy, and immunotherapy.

2. A prospective comparative clinical trial to test the usefulness of subcutaneous mastectomy with augmentation for a specific set of possible precancerous or non-invasive cancers seems justified at this time. The development of more information

about relative risks will be helpful in establishing appropriate criteria for this operative approach.

3. In the future, operative ablation may be helpful in making chemotherapy and immunotherapy more successful and vice versa.

4. The answers to the relative value of operation and radiotherapy alone and in combination for localized and regional mammary cancer can only be determined by prospective comparative clinical trials with careful preselection of groups tested. Unfortunately, resolution of these questions alone will not provide a large number of additional cures.

5. At the present time a reasonable case can be made for the following management of mammary carcinomas in stages A and B [1], without clinical evidence of disseminated disease:

a) Modified radical mastectomy (including removal of pectoralis minor) for lateral lesions without clinical evidence of axillary metastases.

b) Modified radical mastectomy and irradiation through internal mammary and supraclavicular high axillary ports [2] postoperatively for medial and central lesions and those with proved axillary metastases.

c) Irradiation through mammary, internal mammary, and supraclavicular high axillary ports [2] before modified radical mastectomy for the patient with breast badly disturbed by previous surgical intervention.

d) Subcutaneous mastectomy and augmentation, usually bilateral, in patients with lobular carcinoma *in situ,* noninvasive intraductal carcinoma, and precancerous lesions in patients at high risk.

6. Simple mastectomy is indicated at the discretion of the radiotherapist for reducing the mass of tissue to be treated in advanced disease amenable to irradiation.

7. An occasional patient with prolonged survival after having primary neoplasm controlled but with metastatic focus localized in the lung may be cured by resection.

References

1. ACKERMAN, L. V., DEL REGATO, J. A.: Cancer—Diagnosis, Treatment and Prognosis, 2nd edition. St. Louis: The C. V. Mosby Company 1954, p. 1014.
2. AUCHINCLOSS, H.: Significance of Location and Number of Axillary Metastases in Carcinoma of the Breast: A Justification for a Conservative Operation. Ann. Surg. 158, 37 (1963).
3. BRINKLEY, D., HAYBITTLE, J. L.: Treatment of Stage II Carcinoma of the Female Breast. Lancet 2, 291 (1966).
4. BRUCE, Sir J.: Operable Cancer of the Breast. A Controlled Clinical Trial. Cancer (Philad.) 28, 1443—1452 (1971).
5. BUTCHER, H. J., JR., SEAMAN, W. B., ECKERT, C., SALTZSTEIN, S.: An Assessment of Radical Mastectomy and Postoperative Irradiation Therapy in the Treatment of Mammary Cancer. Cancer (Philad.) 17, 480 (1964).
6. CACERES, E.: An Evaluation of Extended Radical Mastectomy in the Treatment of Breast Cancer. In: Breast Cancer: Early and Late, A Collection of Papers Presented at the Thirteenth Annual Clinical Conference on Cancer, 1968 at The University of Texas M. D. Anderson Hospital and Tumor Institute at Houston, Houston, Texas. Chicago: Year Book Medical Publishers, Inc. 1970, pp. 125—134.

---

[1] Columbia Clinical Classification.

[2] Posterior port may be added when necessary.

7. DAHL-IVERSEN, E., TOBIASSEN, T.: Radical Mastectomy with Parasternal and Supra-clavicular Dissection for Mammary Carcinoma. Ann. Surg. 157, 170 (1963).
8. DEN BESTEN. L., ZIFFREN, S. E.: Simple and Radical Mastectomy: A Comparison of Survival. Arch. Surg. 90, 755 (1965).
9. DEVITT, J. E., BEATTIE, W. G.: Rational Treatment of Carcinoma of the Breast? Ann. Surg. 160, 71 (1964).
10. DODD, G. D.: Mammography and Thermography in the Diagnosis of Breast Cancer. In: Breast Cancer: Early and Late, A Collection of Papers Presented at the Thirteenth Annual Clinical Conference on Cancer, 1968 at The University of Texas M. D. Anderson Hospital and Tumor Institute at Houston, Houston, Texas. Chicago: Year Book Medical Publishers, Inc. 1970, pp. 77—88.
11. EGAN, R. L.: Contributions of Mammography in the Detection of Early Breast Cancer. Cancer (Philad.) 28, 1555—1557 (1971).
12. FELLER, W. F., CHOPRA, H. C.: Virus-like Particles in Human Milk. Cancer (Philad.) 28, 1425—1430 (1971).
13. FISHER, B.: The Surgical Dilemma in the Primary Therapy of Invasive Breast Cancer: A Critical Appraisal. In: Current Problems in Surgery. Chicago: Year Book Medical Publishers, Inc., 1970, p. 53.
14. FISHER, B., MOORE, G. E., RAVDIN, R. G., AUSMAN, R. K., SLACK, N. H., NOER, R. J. (and Cooperating Investigators): Surgical Adjuvant Chemotherapy in the Treatment of Breast Cancer. In: Breast Cancer: Early and Late, A Collection of Papers Presented at the Thirteenth Annual Clinical Conference on Cancer, 1968 at The University of Texas M. D. Anderson Hospital and Tumor Institute at Houston, Houston, Texas. Chicago: Year Book Medical Publishers, Inc. 1970, pp. 405—438.
15. FISHER, B., RAVDIN, R. G., AUSMAN, R. K., SLACK, N. H., MOORE, G. E., NOER, R. J. (and Cooperating Investigators): Surgical Adjuvant Chemotherapy in Cancer of the Breast: Results of a Decade of Cooperative Investigation. Ann. Surg. 168(3), 337—356 (1968).
16. FISHER, B., SLACK, N. H., BROSS, I. D. J. (and Cooperating Investigators): Cancer of the Breast: Size of Neoplasm and Prognosis. Cancer (Philad.) 24, 39 (1969).
17. FISHER, B., SLACK, N. H., CAVANAUGH, P. J., GARDNER, G., RAVDIN, R. G. (and Cooperating Investigators): Postoperative Radiotherapy in the Treatment of Breast Cancer: Results of the NSABP Clinical Trial. Ann. Surg. 172, (1970).
18. FLETCHER, G. H.: Local Results of Irradiation in the Primary Management of Localized Breast Cancer. Cancer (Philad.) 29, 545—551 (1972).
19. FREEMAN, B. S.: Subcutaneous Mastectomy for Benign Breast Lesions with Immediate or Delayed Prosthetic Replacement. Plast. reconstr. Surg. 30, 676—682 (1962).
20. GALLAGER, H. S., MARTIN, J. E.: An Orientation to the Concept of Minimal Breast Cancer. Cancer (Philad.) 28, 1505—1507 (1971).
21. HAAGENSEN, C. D.: Carcinoma of the Breast in Its Earlier Stages. In: Breast Cancer: Early and Late, A Collection of Papers Presented at the Thirteenth Annual Clinical Conference on Cancer, 1968 at The University of Texas M. D. Anderson Hospital and Tumor Institute at Houston, Houston, Texas. Chicago: Year Book Medical Publishers, Inc. 1970, pp. 405—438.
22. HAAGENSEN, C. D., COOLEY, E.: Radical Mastectomy for Mammary Carcinoma. Ann. Surg. 170, 884 (1969).
23. HAAGENSEN, C. D., COOLEY, E., KENNEDY, C. S., MILLER, E., HANDLEY, R. S., THACKRAY, A. C., BUTCHER, H. R., JR., DAHL-IVERSEN, E., TOBIASSEN, T., WILLIAMS, I. G., CURWEN, M. P., KAAE, S., JOHANSEN, H.: Treatment of Early Mammary Carcinoma. A Cooperative International Study. Ann. Surg. 157, 157 (1963).
24. HAAGENSEN, C. D., MILLER, E.: Is Radical Mastectomy the Optimal Procedure for Early Breast Carcinoma? J. Amer. Med. Ass. 199, 739 (1967).
25. HAAGENSEN, C. D., STOUT, A. P.: Carcinoma of the Breast. II. Criteria of Operability. Ann. Surg. 118, 859 and continued 1032 (1943).
26. HALSTED, W. S.: The Treatment of Wounds. IV. Operations for Carcinoma of the Breast. Surgical Papers 1, 87, The Johns Hopkins Press, Baltimore, Maryland, 1922. Johns Hopk. Hosp. Rep. 2, 255 (1890—1891).

27. Halsted, W. S.: The Results of Operations for the Cure of Cancer of the Breast Performed at the Johns Hopkins Hospital from June, 1889 to January, 1894. Johns Hopk. Hosp. Rep. 4, 297 (1894—1895).

28. Halsted, W. S.: A Clinical and Histological Study of Certain Adenocarcinomas of the Breast and a Brief Consideration of the Supraclavicular Operation and of the Results of Operations for Cancer of the Breast from 1889 to 1898 at the Johns Hopkins Hospital. Ann. Surg. 28, 144 (1898).

29. Halsted, W. S.: The Results of Radical Operations for the Cure of Carcinoma of the Breast. Ann. Surg. 46, 1 (1907).

30. Handley, R. S.: The Early Spread of Breast Carcinoma and its Bearing on Operative Treatment. Brit. J. Surg. 51, 206 (1964).

31. Handley, R. S.: The Technic and Results of Conservative Radical Mastectomy (Patey's Operation). Progr. Clin. Cancer 1, 462 (1965).

32. Handley, R. S., Thackray, A. C.: Invasion of the Internal Mammary Lymph Glands in Carcinoma of the Breast. Brit. J. Cancer 1, 15 (1947).

33. Healey, J. E., Jr.: Cancer of the Breast: The Role of Rehabilitation. In: Progress in the Rehabilitation of the Cancer Patient, A Collection of Papers Presented at the Fifteenth Annual Clinical Conference at The University of Texas M. D. Anderson Hospital and Tumor Institute at Houston, Houston, Texas. Chicago: Year Book Medical Publishers, Inc. In press 1972.

34. Hepner, G.: In Breast Cancer, is There Evidence That Immunity Influences Tumor Host Balance? In: Breast Cancer: A Challenging Problem. In press 1972.

35. Hoerr, S. O.: Local Excision for Carcinoma of the Breast: Its Possible Use in Special Situations. Amer. J. Surg. 109, 399 (1965).

36. Hutter, R. V. P., Foote, F. W., Jr., Farrow, J. H.: In Situ Lobular Carcinoma of the Female Breast, 1939—1968. In: Breast Cancer: Early and Late, A Collection of Papers Presented at the Thirteenth Annual Clinical Conference on Cancer, 1968 at The University of Texas M. D. Anderson Hospital and Tumor Institute at Houston, Houston, Texas. Chicago: Year Book Medical Publishers, Inc., 1970, pp. 201—226.

37. Jensen, E.: Hormonal Dependency of Breast Cancer: How is this Factor Clinically Significant? In: Breast Cancer: A Challenging Problem. In press 1972.

38. Kaae, S., Johansen, H.: Simple Mastectomy Plus Postoperative Irradiation by the Method of McWhirter for Mammary Carcinoma. Progr. Clin. Cancer 1, 453 (1965).

39. Kennedy, C. S., Miller, E.: Simple Mastectomy for Mammary Carcinoma. Ann. Surg. 157, 161—162 (1963).

40. Madden, J. L.: Modified Radical Mastectomy. Surg. Gynec. Obstet. 121, 1221 (1965).

41. McWhirter, R.: The Value of Simple Mastectomy and Radiotherapy in the Treatment of Cancer of the Breast. Brit. J. Radiol. 21, 599 (1948).

42. Mendelsohn, M.: Implications of Normal Tissue and Breast Cancer Cell Kinetics in Breast Cancer Management. In: Breast Cancer: A Challenging Problem. In press 1972.

43. Mustakallio, S.: Treatment of Breast Cancer by Tumor Extirpation and Roentgen Therapy Instead of Radical Operation. J. Fac. Radiol. (Lond.) 6, 23 (1954).

44. Nissen-Meyer, R.: Is Prophylactic Use of Hormonal Therapy Beneficial in the Outcome of Breast Cancer? In: Breast Cancer: A Challenging Problem. In press 1972.

45. Patey, D. H., Dyson, W. H.: The Prognosis of Carcinoma of the Breast in Relation to the Type of Operation Performed. Brit. J. Cancer 2, 7 (1948).

46. Peters, M. V.: The Role of Local Excision and Radiation in Early Breast Cancer. In: Breast Cancer: Early and Late, A Collection of Papers Presented at the Thirteenth Annual Clinical Conference on Cancer, 1968 at The University of Texas M. D. Anderson Hospital and Tumor Institute at Houston, Houston, Texas. Chicago: Year Book Medical Publishers, Inc., 1970, pp. 171—189.

47. Petrakis, N. L., Pingle, U., Petrakis, S. J., Petrakis, S. L.: Evidence for a Genetic Cline in Ear Wax Types in the Middle East and Southeast Asia. Amer. J. Phys. Anthrop. 35, 141—144 (1971).

48. Porritt, A.: Early Carcinoma of the Breast. Brit. J. Surg. 51, 214 (1964).

49. RAVDIN, R. G., LEWISON, E. F., SLACK, N. H., DAO, T. L., GARDNER, B., STATE, D., FISHER, B. (and Cooperating Investigators): The Worth of Prophylactic Oöphorectomy in the Treatment of Operable Breast Cancer: Results of the NSABP Clinical Trial. Surg. Gynec. Obstet. 131, (1970).
50. RAVENTOS, A.: Postoperative Radiation Therapy. Cancer (Philad.) 28, 1651—1653 (1971).
51. RAVITCH, M. M.: Carcinoma of the Breast. The Place of the Halsted Radical Mastectomy. Choice of Operation for Breast Cancer. Cancer (Philad.) 129, 202—211 (1971).
52. SPIEGELMAN, S., SCHLOM, J.: Molecular Probes for the Viral Etiology of Human Breast Cancer. In: Molecular Studies in Viral Neoplasia. In press 1972.
53. URBAN, J. A.: Bilateral Breast Cancer. In: Breast Cancer: Early and Late, A Collection of Papers Presented at the Thirteenth Annual Clinical Conference on Cancer, 1968 at The University of Texas M. D. Anderson Hospital and Tumor Institute at Houston, Houston, Texas. Chicago: Year Book Medical Publishers, Inc., 1970, pp. 263—272.
54. URBAN, J. A., CASTRO, E. B.: Selecting Variations in Extent of Surgical Procedure for Breast Cancer. Cancer (Philad.) 28, 1615—1623 (1971).
55. VERONESI, U., ZINGO, L.: Extended Mastectomy for Cancer of the Breast. Cancer (Philad.) 20, 677 (1967).
56. WANGENSTEEN, O. H., LEWIS, F. J.: Radical Mastectomy with Dissection of Supraclavicular Mediastinal and Internal Mammary Lymph Nodes. In: Treatment of Cancer and Allied Diseases, Second Edition. Eds.: G. T. PACK and I. M. ARIEL. 4, 122. P. B. Hoeber, Inc. 1960, Vol. 4, p. 122.
57. WATSON, T. A.: Treatment of Breast Cancer: Comparison of Results of Simple Mastectomy and Radiotherapy with Results of Radical Mastectomy and Radiotherapy. Lancet 1959 I, 1191.
58. WHITE, E. C.: Selection of Treatment for Patients with Potentially Curable Cancer of the Breast. In: Breast Cancer: Early and Late, A Collection of Papers Presented at the Thirteenth Annual Clinical Conference on Cancer, 1968 at The University of Texas M. D. Anderson Hospital and Tumor Institute at Houston, Houston, Texas. Chicago: Year Book Medical Publishers, Inc. 1970, pp. 155—160.
59. WILLIAMS, J. G., MURLEY, R. S., CURWEN, M. P.: Carcinoma of the Female Breast: Conservative Radical Surgery. Brit. Med. J. 2, 787 (1953).
60. WYNDER, E. L.: Identification of Women at High Risk for Breast Cancer. Cancer (Philad.) 24, 1235—1240 (1969).
61. ZIPPIN, C., PETRAKIS, N. L.: Identification of High Risk Groups in Breast Cancer. Cancer (Philad.) 28, 1381—1387 (1971).

Is Prophylactic Use of Hormonal Therapy or Cytostatic Chemotherapy Beneficial in the Outcome of Breast Cancer?

R. Nissen-Meyer

During recent years, several randomized clinical trials have been published, comparing various modifications of the primary treatment for breast cancer. Some of these series could not demonstrate that the treatment modality under study had any significant influence on the outcome of the disease. The consequence has been a general tendency towards a less radical primary treatment, but some clinicians wonder if this tendency is sound.

In trials designed to study effect of the primary treatment on disease-free interval and survival, we randomize a series of patients clinically classified as primary, operable cases. We may try to subdivide the series, mostly into stage I (axillary nodes negative) and stage II (axillary nodes positive), but in fact the patients will belong to a wide variety of subgroup combinations. Some of the more obvious subgroups are shown in Fig. 1. The place of one particular patient in this system may only be roughly estimated clinically.

An improvement of one particular part of the total treatment scheme may improve the results in one particular combination of these subgroups. For example, the

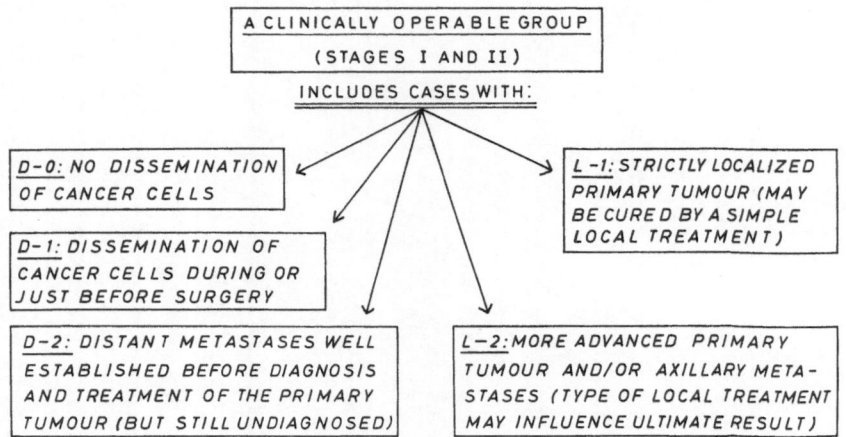

Fig. 1

radicality of the local treatment (surgery and local irradiation) will only influence the results in the combination L-2 and D-0 in Fig. 1. Statistically, even a definite improvement in such a small part of the total mass of patients may easily be diluted by the unaltered results in all the other patients and escape our observation. This makes it necessary to randomize a large number of patients and sometimes look for rather small differences in the total results.

Furthermore, the nature of the improvement obtained with one method may be completely different from that obtained with another. An endocrine treatment may not cure any patient, only reduce the growth rate of the remaining tumour tissue, and result in an average increase of the free interval. Adjuvant chemotherapy, on the other hand, may be expected to reduce the number of recurrences, and we believe especially of the late recurrences. This makes it necessary to look specifically for that kind of effect we may suppose to get with the treatment modality in question and to look for it in the groups of patients most likely to respond.

In the following pages, we will describe two controlled clinical trials designed to study the effect of primary castration and of adjuvant chemotherapy.

A. Primary Castration

The only intention of primary castration is to delay the course of the cancer, to give the patients a longer interval free of clinical disease before their metastases have developed to a size giving distressing symptoms, and possibly, also to prolong their remaining time of life. The patients benefitting from this adjuvant treatment are of course only those carrying viable cancer cells. We cannot, however, treat these patients without also treating a number of patients who were already definitely cured by the primary treatment and for whom the additional endocrine treatment is an unnecessary burden. This makes it necessary earnestly to consider the risk and side effects of the treatment in relation to the risk of the disease itself.

To a certain degree we can estimate the risk that a patient belongs to the group with subclinical metastases. A large tumour, involvement of the axillary nodes, localization to the inner quadrants of the breast, and a high malignancy grading make it more likely that local recurrences or distant metastases will develop.

The easiest way to study the effect of primary castration would have been to randomize the high-risk premenopausal patients between a castration group and a control group. However, randomizing such patients to a control group would meet with strong ethical objections if the investigator feels it most probable that the majority of them might benefit from the treatment.

A study was therefore designed, being a sort of compromize between the statistician's desire for an optimal statistical evaluation and the clinician's wish to treat each patient individually according to the best of his knowledge. The principle was that only borderline cases should be randomized, cases where doubt existed about the best choice, taking into consideration the prognosis of the disease, the possible effect of the treatment and the risk and side effects of this treatment.

During the 6-year period from 22. November 1957 to 31. December 1963, all histologically verified cases of breast cancer admitted to The Norwegian Radium Hospital were registered for a prospective study of the effect of endocrine treatment. A total of 1129 patients were classified as stage I and II, and formed the case material

for a study of primary (socalled "prophylactic") *versus* "therapeutic" castration. The
primary endocrine treatment was as follows: 605 patients received primary ovarian
irradiation (a total dose of 1000 r to each ovary, given during 6 days), whereas primary ovariectomy was performed in 74 patients. The rest, 450 patients, had no primary castration, but castration was planned to be performed as soon as possible if
recurrences were diagnosed. If recurrences were diagnosed, prednisone treatment
(2.5 mg four times daily) was also given, in order to suppress pituitary-adreno-
cortical function.

According to the principles discussed above, 448 out of the 1129 patients were
included in controlled clinical trial series with random allocation between treatment
groups.

In a previous publication [1] full details are given about the composition of the
groups of patients discussed in the present paper, as well as about the treatment
methods, the criteria, and the statistical methods used.

The questions were:

1. Does castration as adjunct to mastectomy give an increased interval free of
symptoms in the patients not cured by mastectomy; and in case it does, how much is
it increased?

2. Is the total survival longer with primary castration than it is with a policy of
"therapeutic" castration?

3. Is there any effect of castration in postmenopausal women?

4. Is ovariectomy more effective for this purpose than ovarian irradiation?

Results

One hundred and sixty-one premenopausal patients with a favourable prognosis
were randomized between primary ovarian irradiation and no primary castration
(Fig. 2). The results are in favour of the treatment group, both in terms of disease-free
intervals and rates of crude survival. The difference in rates free of disease is now
significant with $P < 0.05$. The difference in survival rates is not significant yet.

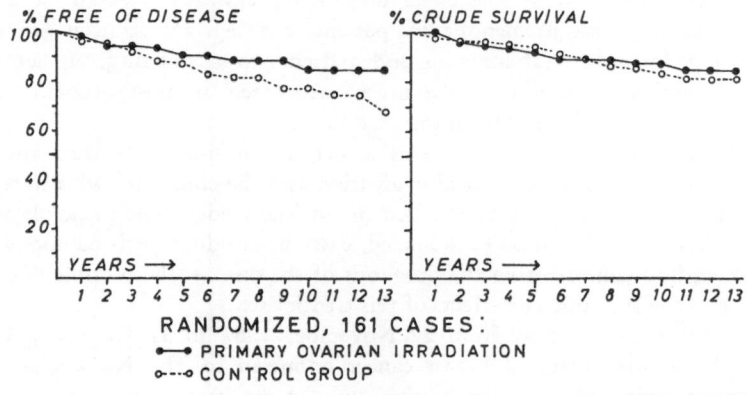

PREMENOPAUSAL, LOW-RISK

RANDOMIZED, 161 CASES:
●—● PRIMARY OVARIAN IRRADIATION
o---o CONTROL GROUP

FEBRUARY 1972

Fig. 2

One hundred and seventy-five postmenopausal patients (average age 60 years) were also randomized between primary ovarian irradiation and no primary castration (Fig. 3). The results were significantly in favour of the treatment group, both in terms of disease-free intervals and rates of crude survival, both in Stage I and in Stage II. These somewhat surprising results are supported by the finding that urinary oestrone

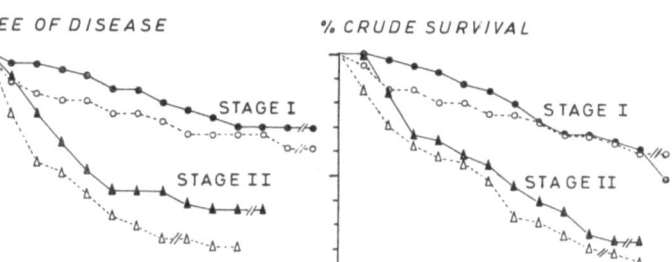

Fig. 3

Table. Estimate of average gain per patient not cured by mastectomy in the Oslo series and the Manchester series [a]. Primary ovarian irradiation versus control

	Cases in series	Follow-up	Years free of symptoms	Total years of live
Premenopausal:				
Low-risk series, Oslo	161	12 years	2.83	0.43
Stage I, Manchester	195	15 years	3.02	
Stage II, Manchester	403	15 years	2.29	
Postmenopausal:				
Stage I, Oslo	80	12 years	3.00	1.63
Stage II, Oslo	95	10 years	1.84	1.06

[a] The Manchester series according to Dr. M. P. COLE 1972.

excretion continues for many years after menopause, and is suppressed by the ovarian irradiation [2, 3, 4].

The table summarizes the estimated average gain in years free of symptoms and years total life per patient not cured by the primary treatment. Included in this Table are also the results from the corresponding clinical trials at The Christie Hospital in Manchester, by kind permission of Dr. MARY P. COLE [4, 5, 6]. The average gain obtained by primary ovarian irradiation seems to be in the order of 2—3 years added to the free interval. It should be unnecessary to emphasize that if a patient is not cured by the mastectomy, but deemed to get recurrences and die from her cancer, the disease-free interval is the most valuable part of her remaining lifetime.

An analysis of the results in the non-randomized cases of the total series of 1129 patients from The Norwegian Radium Hospital [1, 3] supports the results found in the randomized series.

One hundred and twelve premenopausal high-risk patients were randomized between primary ovarian irradiation and primary ovariectomy (Fig. 4). Much to our surprise the results were in favour of the ovarian irradiated group, but the difference

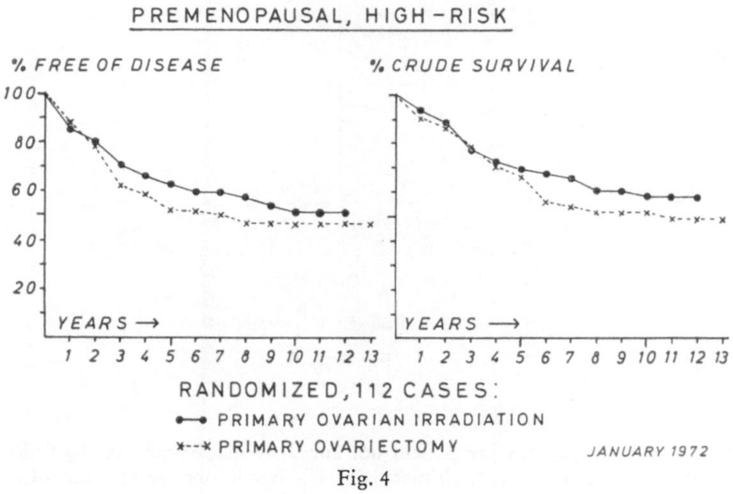

PREMENOPAUSAL, HIGH—RISK

Fig. 4

is not statistically significant. The difference may therefore be due to chance, but theoretically it may also be possible that irradiation may alter the enzyme system of the ovaries in a way that makes this treatment more favourable for such cases than a surgical removal of the ovaries. One can easily imagine that after ovarian irradiation the hormone profile may be changed, for example, to a more favourable oestriol/oestrone + oestradiol ratio [cfr. 7] or that some ovarian factors are left for suppression of tumour-stimulating pituitary factors. There is much left for research in this field.

B. Adjuvant Chemotherapy

There are cases which never get metastases and are cured when the primary tumour is removed. We also know that there are cases with subclinical (undiagnosed) metastases firmly established at their new site of growth and with a considerable size before the primary tumour is diagnosed and treated. Logically, then there must also exist at least some cases which have their first dissemination and "takes" of cancer cells during surgery or during the preceeding days with diagnostic procedures. When we consider the often very rough handling of the primary tumour during these procedures, one would suspect that this group is not so small.

We know that we cannot eradicate completely diagnosed metastases from breast cancer with any of the cytostatic drugs now available. We do not believe that this may be possible if the metastases are subclinical, but well established before the primary tumour is removed. We have some hope, however, that a total eradication of the cancer cells might be achieved if these were quite recently disseminated from the primary tumour and not firmly established at their new site. I shall report a controlled clinical trial performed in a number of cooperating centers in Finland, Sweden and Norway as an attempt to assess this possibility. The set-up of the trial and the

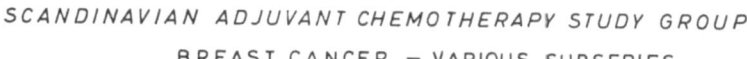

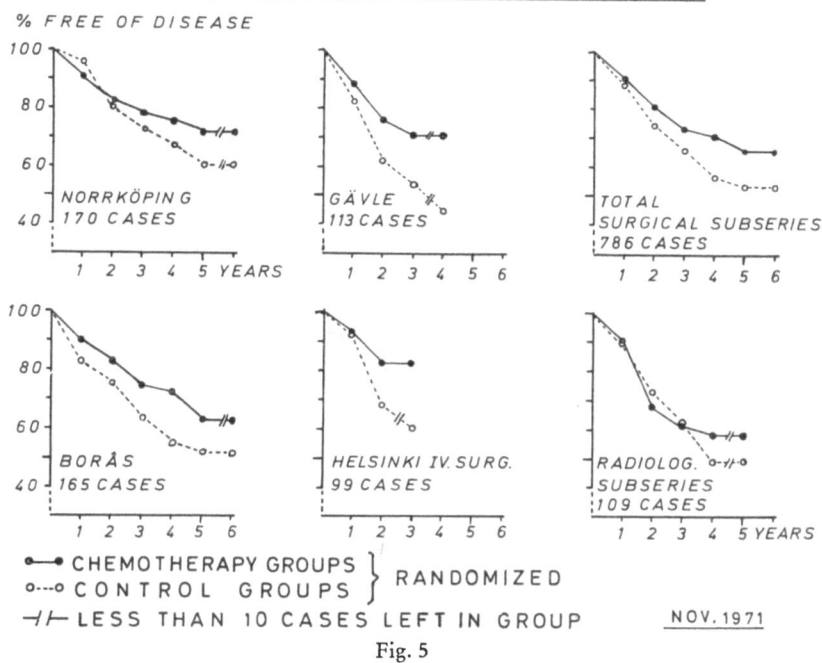

Fig. 5

preliminary results as of April 1970 has already been published [8]. The drug given was cyclophosphamide; the total dose 30 mg/kg body weight was given during 6 days.

The main point in our hypothesis is the assumption that growth from one disseminated breast cancer cell to a clinically detectable metastasis usually takes more than two years. (This may be deducted from a number of studies of the net volume doubling time of breast cancer both in man and animal.) This means that we cannot expect that one short postoperative course of chemotherapy should influence the results during the first few years after surgery, but we did hope that the number of late-occurring recurrences should be diminished.

The following is a report of the results as of November 1971. Until May 1971 we had randomized 895 cases. In the control group 142 recurrences were registered, in the chemotherapy group only 98 recurrences. The difference of 44 recurrences is statistically significant with a P value of < 0.01. In the control group 93 deaths were recorded, in the chemotherapy group 78. This difference in deaths is not statistically significant as yet, but the difference will probably increase with a longer follow-up time, in view of the larger difference in recurrences already noted.

Fig. 5 shows the results from some of the hospitals which have already reported about 100 cases or more, as well as the results in the total surgical subseries (chemotherapy given immediately after surgery) and in the radiological subseries (chemotherapy given during postoperative local irradiation, about three weeks after surgery). It may be seen that in all subseries the outcome is better in the treatment group, and the difference between the two groups increases with increasing follow-up time after surgery. These findings are in complete harmony with our hypothesis. In the total surgical subseries the difference reaches statistical significance with P < 0.01 four years after surgery.

In Fig. 6 the total material is split up into stage I (axillary nodes negative) and stage II (axillary nodes positive). In both stages there is a difference in favour of the

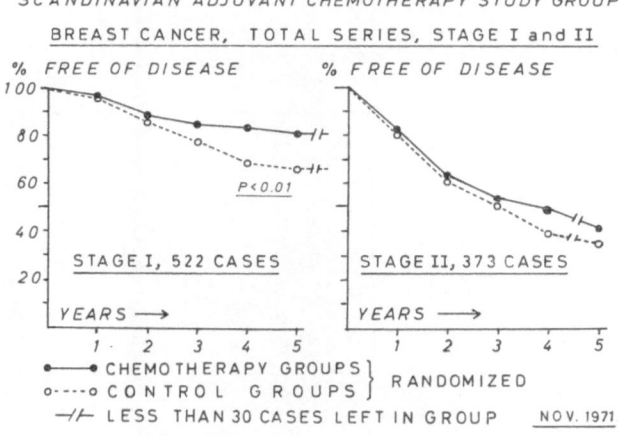

Fig. 6

chemotherapy group, but the difference is most pronounced in stage I, where it again reaches a statistical significance with P < 0.01 four years after surgery.

This observation, that the best effect was obtained in stage I cases, fits also very well with the hypothesis that a short course of adjuvant chemotherapy will only eradicate the newly disseminated cancer cells and not the older subclinical metastases, well established before surgery. It seems quite logical to assume that the patients, who had no distant metastases until handling of the primary tumour during diagnostic procedures and surgery brought about a dissemination of cancer cells, are more frequent in stage I.

This latter observation implies that chemotherapy should not mainly be used as a supplement to surgery in cases with locally advanced primary tumours and large axillary nodes, as it seems to be the policy in many clinics. On the contrary, the main advantage of adjuvant chemotherapy seems to be that it can make the good prognosis in early clinically localized cases still better.

Summary

Controlled clinical studies have shown that primary ovarian irradiation significantly increases the disease-free interval after mastectomy. This increase is at an average 2—3 years, both in premenopausal and postmenopausal cases. The total survival time was also increased compared with the groups with "therapeutic" castration after diagnosis of recurrences. Surgical ovariectomy was not found to be better than ovarian irradiation.

Adjuvant chemotherapy (cyclophosphamide, total dose 30 mg/kg, given intravenously during 6 days) reduced significantly the number of recurrences diagnosed 3 or more years after mastectomy. This effect seemed to be best in stage I cases.

References

1. NISSEN-MEYER, R.: Castration as part of the primary treatment for operable female breast cancer. A statistical evaluation of clinical results. Acta radiol. (Stockh.) Suppl. 249 (1965).
2. NISSEN-MEYER, R., SANNER, T.: The excretion of oestrone, pregnanediol and pregnanetriol in breast cancer patients. I. Excretion after spontaneous menopause. Acta endocr. (Kbh.) 44, 325 (1963).
3. NISSEN-MEYER, R., SANNER, T.: The excretion of oestrone, pregnanediol and pregnanetriol in breast cancer patients. II. Effects of ovariectomy, ovarian irradiation and corticosteroids. Acta endocr. (Kbh.) 44, 334 (1963).
4. NISSEN-MEYER, R.: The role of prophylactic castration in the therapy of human mammary cancer. Europ. J. Cancer 3, 395 (1967).
5. COLE, M. P.: Suppression of ovarian function in primary breast cancer. In: Prognostic Factors in Breast Cancer. Eds.: FORREST, A. P. M., KUNKLER, P. B. Baltimore: The Williams and Wilkins Company 1968, p. 146.
6. COLE, M. P.: Personal communication, 1972.
7. COLE, P., MACMAHON, B.: Oestrogen fractions during early reproductive life in the aetiology of breast cancer. Lancet 1969 I, 604.
8. NISSEN-MEYER, R., KJELLGREN, K., MÅNSSON, B.: Preliminary report from the Scandinavian Adjuvant Chemotherapy Study Group. Cancer Chemother. Reports 55, 561 (1971).

The Role of Hormone Therapy in the Management of Metastatic Breast Cancer

T. L. Dao

Appreciation of the results of the investigation of Huggins and his co-workers on tumors of the prostate [1] led to an intensive search for effective hormonal therapy in many forms of human cancers, including those of the mammary gland. The control of neoplasia, either by removal of hormonal factors (sources) or by administration of hormones, represents a challenging area of research which has real clinical implications. Unfortunately endocrine control of metastatic breast cancer is often transient and is limited to only a small number of patients, while in the majority of cases the disease is affected only slightly or not at all.

The endocrine control of breast cancer rests upon the alteration of the host endocrine environment or hormonal millieu through the eradication of hormonal sources or the administration of steroid hormones. The lack of significant progress in the treatment of breast cancer by hormonal methods is due largely to our ignorance in the understanding of the mechanism by which hormones control normal and neoplastic mammary glands.

Control of Advanced Breast Cancer by Steroid Hormones

Estrogen has been shown to induce mammary cancer in both mice and rats. The use of androgenic hormones in the treatment of human breast cancer began after the experiments of Lacassagne [2] and Nathanson and Andervont [3] showed that androgen could prevent induction of breast cancer by estrogen in mice. It is believed that the anti-neoplastic activity of androgen in mammary cancer is due to its anti-estrogenic activity. The exact mechanism by which androgen induces regression of advanced breast cancer, however, is not clearly understood.

To date, hormonal steroids including androgens, estrogens, progestins, and adrenocorticosteroids have all been used in the treatment of advanced breast cancer. This author will not provide any detailed review in this paper. Readers may refer to a review article to be published in 1973 [4]. It appears that steroid hormones have little specificity in inducing regression of breast cancer, since nearly all of them show some effectiveness, even though they possess very different biological activities. For an example, estrogen is anti-androgenic, but it causes tumor regression in some women with breast cancer. Paradoxically, estrogen has been shown to accelerate mammary cancer growth in some women.

The most widely used hormonal steroids in the treatment of breast cancer are the androgens, estrogens, and adrenocorticoids. There is little evidence to indicate that either sequential use or cross-over administration of these hormones produces additional benefits to patients with advanced breast cancer. Often patients who fail to respond to one hormone are equally refractory to the others. In rare instances, however, patients responding to one hormone and in relapse, may derive further palliative benefit from another hormone with very different biological activities.

The anti-tumor efficacy of androgens and estrogens are similar. They benefit about 20% of the patients with disseminated breast cancer. These compounds induce regression mainly of the soft tissue lesions and osseous metastases. It is only rarely that one observes the regression of visceral metastases in women treated either with testosterone or estrogen. The usual clinical practice of using estrogen in older women and testesterone in younger patients is not based on scientific evidence. The age of the patient is not a criterion for choosing either androgen or estrogen in the treatment of advanced breast cancer. In fact, testosterone is as effective in older patients as is in younger women with advanced breast cancer. The clinicians who use androgens and estrogens must be aware of the side effects of these hormones which may be fatal to patients with advanced breast cancer. Of particular importance are the effects of these hormones in causing hypercalcemia, alterations of salt and water metabolism and psychological disturbances in older women as a result of increased sexual libido and virilizing symptoms following testosterone therapy.

The use of adrenal corticosteroid hormones in the treatment of advanced breast cancer perhaps deserves some special mention. The impressive clinical results of adrenalectomy in women with advanced breast cancer led to the use of adrenal corticosteroids in an attempt to suppress adrenocortical activity sufficiently to induce a similar tumor regression. Objective tumor regression in cancer of the breast following large doses of cortisone occurs in about 20—30% of the patients. The most commonly used compound now is Prednisone. Adrenal corticoid therapy, however, cannot reproduce the definitive regression observed in patients following adrenalectomy. It must be mentioned that the toxicities as a result of corticosteroid therapy can be serious, particularly those concerned with the electrolyte and carbohydrate metabolism.

Ablation Therapy for Disseminated Breast Cancer

Although excision of endocrine glands to control human breast cancer was first introduced by BEATSON in 1896 [5], bilateral oophorectomy was not widely performed until the late 1940's. The early 1950's witnessed the introduction of adrenalectomy [6] and hypophysectomy [7] for the treatment of breast cancer. The endocrine ablation therapy in breast cancer has been reviewed recently in detail by this author [8].

Castration performed as a palliative measure in women with advanced breast cancer is effective in about 30% of premenopausal women so treated. In hormone-dependent breast cancer, visceral metastases as well as soft tissue and osseous metastases will regress after oophorectomy. It should be emphasized that the beneficial effects of castration are essentially confined to premenopausal women. Although castration may occasionally be of value a few years after menopause, the operation is not justified unless there is definite evidence of significant residual ovarian activities. In a series of 202 consecutive cases, we observed that incidence of remission was

significantly lower when castration was performed in menopausal women and none
in postmenopausal patients (Fig. 1). The data clearly indicate that one cannot justify
surgical castration in postmenopausal women with advanced cancer of the breast.

The poor results of mastectomy in young women with breast cancer and the
apparent benefits of castration in some women with disseminated breast cancer led to
the empirical use of castration at the time of mastectomy to improve the cure rate.
Although NISSEN-MEYER has demonstrated an increase in survival rate in all patients

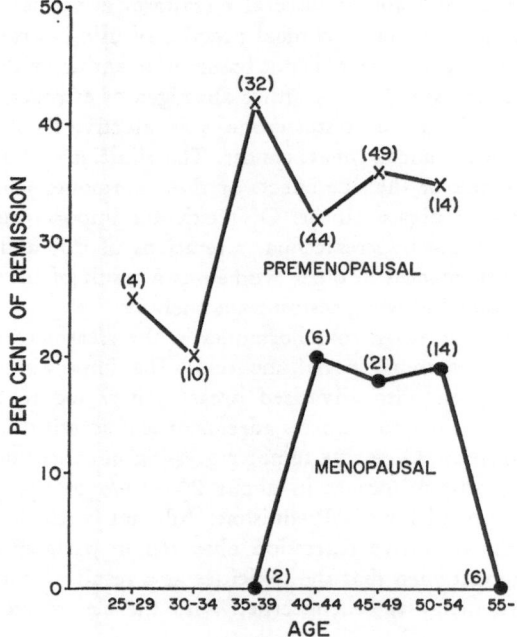

Fig. 1. Age and menopausal status in relation to response to castration in women with metastatic cancer of the breast. Number of patients in each group indicated in parentheses

who underwent prophylactic castration at the time of "curative" mastectomy, similar
results were not obtained by a prospective study carried out by the National Surgical
Adjuvant Breast Group in the U.S.A. [9]. Our data (Tables 1 and 2) show that there
is no difference at any time, in either the recurrence or survival rate, between patients
undergoing prophylactic castration and those in the control group. When patients
were classified according to the status of adjacent lymph nodes, i. e., positive or
negative for cancer content, no advantage was obtained for patients after castration.
It perhaps is a wise policy to withhold oophorectomy until recurrence appears, for
the following reasons: (a) lack of conclusive evidence to support the supposition that
prophylactic castration can either reduce recurrence rate or prolong survival; (b) induction of menopausal symptoms as a result of castration which is detrimental to the
patient; and (c) the fact that favorable response to castration in patients with
advanced breast cancer frequently is followed by favorable response to adrenalectomy or hypophysectomy.

Table 1. Recurrence rates for patients with negative and positive nodes

Mos. after operation	Oophorectomy			Controls		
	No.	No. recur- rences	% recur- rences	No.	No. recur- rences	% recur- rences
Negative nodes						
12	58	2	3	85	4	5
18	57	5	9	80	7	9
24	56	7	12	72	7	10
30	49	10	20	70	10	14
36	48	10	21	67	11	16
Positive nodes						
12	78	21	27	95	25	26
18	73	27	37	92	36	39
24	70	29	41	88	42	48
30	68	34	50	85	45	53
36	67	37	55	78	46	59

Table 2. Survival rate for patients with negative and positive nodes

Mos. after operation	Oophorectomy			Controls		
	No.	No. surviving	% survival	No.	No. surviving	% survival
Negative nodes						
12	58	58	100	85	84	99
18	56	55	98	80	78	98
24	55	51	93	72	69	96
30	48	43	90	70	64	91
36	47	41	87	66	58	88
Positive nodes						
12	78	72	92	93	91	98
18	74	60	81	90	79	88
24	69	49	71	84	67	80
30	66	44	67	78	54	69
36	64	38	59	69	44	64

The question whether "total" suppression of ovarian activity can be achieved by X-ray irradiation cannot be easily answered. It is obvious that surgical castration essentially guarantees the complete eradication of ovarian function. The rapid effect as a result of abrupt removal of ovarian hormones by surgical castration often induces remarkable relief of acute symptoms such as crippling bone pain from osseous metastases and respiratory difficulty from pulmonary metastases.

The introduction of bilateral adrenalectomy represents an important addition to the armamentarium for the treatment of advanced breast cancer [10]. The replacement therapy required has long since been proven safe, and bilateral adrenalectomy is no longer a perilous operation. Adrenalectomized patients, when maintained adequately on cortisone, have a healthy appearance, are not incapacitated, and are able to engage in most of their usual activities.

The clinical results of adrenalectomy have been well established [8]. It is particularly noteworthy that adrenalectomy not only induces regression of soft tissue and bone metastases but that it is equally effective for visceral metastases. A frequent question is whether adrenalectomy should be done as a primary treatment in patients with disseminated breast cancer without first administering hormonal therapy (primary adrenalectomy). We carried out a randomized study to compare the results of primary adrenalectomy vs. secondary adrenalectomy (adrenalectomy after hormonal therapy). The results, published earlier [11], disclose that the objective regression rate is considerably better for primary adrenalectomy (46%) than for secondary adrenalectomy (30%). In that study, we also found that neither response nor lack of response to previous hormonal therapy can be correlated with subsequent response to adrenalectomy. Our results showed that objective remission following adrenalectomy occurred in 30% of the patients who had responded to hormonal therapy and in 37% of the non-responders.

In spite of the noteworthy palliation of advanced breast cancer by adrenalectomy, proper selection of patients for this major surgical procedure is imparative if nonresponsive patients can be spared from an unnecessary major operation. As yet we do not have a laboratory method which can be used to distinguish hormone-responsive from hormone-nonresponsive breast cancer. Recent studies of intracellular macromolecules with high stereospecific affinity for estrogens have revealed the existence of specific protein receptors in estrogen-responsive tissues including the mammary gland [12]. This elegant work of JENSEN et al. has now been extended to both experimental and human breast cancer. The possible clinical correlation between the presence or absence of estrogen receptor protein in the mammary cancer tissue and its response to endocrine ablation is presented by Dr. JENSEN at this symposium.

I wish, however, to report briefly some recent work from my laboratory concerning the capacity of breast tumors to synthesize sulfate esters of steroid hormones. We demonstrated that the breast cancer tissue contained two populations of cells, one that lacked enzyme and one that possessed enzymes capable of forming sulfate esters with several steroid hormones [13]. We also observed that the pattern of conjugation of steriod hormones is not the same in breast cancer tissue as it is in the normal liver tissue. The ability of the breast cancer tissue to conjugate estrogenic and androgenic hormones varies from one individual to another. Some breast cancers have enzyme systems that synthesize estrogen sulfate more efficiently than they do dehydroepiandrosterone sulfate, whereas the case with others may be the reverse.

These findings led to a study to determine whether the formation of steroid sulfates in mammary cancer is related to the response to endocrine ablation in patients with advanced cancer of the breast. We reported earlier [14] that if breast tumors did not possess enzymes for the synthesis of steroid conjugates, they would not regress after adrenalectomy. Breast cancer tissue which synthesizes more dehydroepiandrosterone sulfate than estrogen sulfate regresses after adrenalectomy.

In an extended study, we have further confirmed the earlier data. Table 3 shows data clearly demonstrating the correlation between the results of the *in vitro* study and clinical response to adrenalectomy. Perhaps the most striking observation is the finding that patients whose tumors do not possess sulfotransferases uniformly fail to respond to adrenalectomy, and all are dead (Fig. 2). In contrast, the survival rate in patients having tumors that form more DHEA sulfate than estradiol sulfate is significantly better.

Table 3. Sulfokinase activity in tumor and response to adrenalectomy

No. of patients	Sulfokinase activity in tumor DHEA : E-17β ratio	Response to adrenalectomy	
		Remission	Failure
30	No activity	—	30
46	< 1	6 (15%)	40
29	> 1	21 (73%)	8
4	= 1	3	1
Total 109		30	79

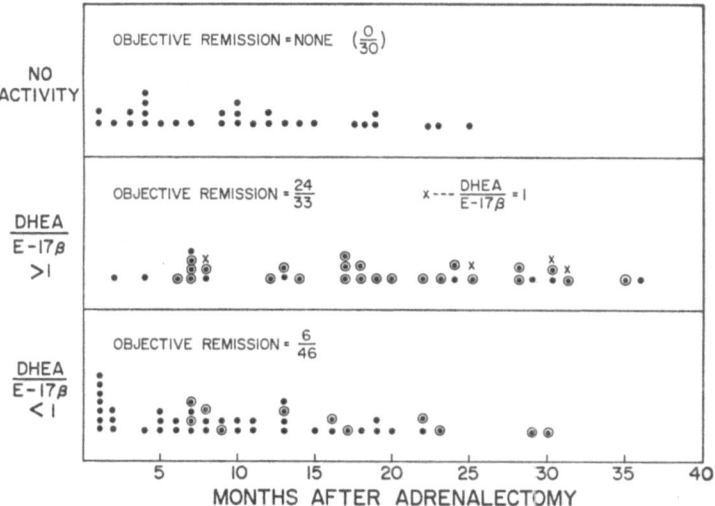

Fig. 2. Correlation between steroid sulfotransferase activity in tumor and survival after adrenalectomy. ⊙ — Living, ● — Dead, × — Living in group with ratio = 1

Conclusion

Although beneficial effects as a result of endocrine alteration in women with advanced breast cancer can be obtained either by administering hormonal steroids or by ablating endocrine glands, all clinical evidence shows that endocrine ablative procedures are therapeutically much more effective than administrative hormonal therapy. Our study discloses that endocrine ablation should be considered as a primary treatment of choice in women with visceral metastasis because hormonal therapy is ineffective. In those patients whose predominant metastases are soft tissue or osseous, hormonal therapy may be considered as primary treatment before adrenalectomy or hypophysectomy.

It has generally been agreed that bilateral oophorectomy should be done as the treatment in all premenopausal women with disseminated breast cancer. Those who obtain objective regression after oophorectomy should be treated either with adrenalectomy or hypophysectomy when disease recurs. In patients who do not respond to oophorectomy, treatment with chemotherapy perhaps is a better choice. It should be emphasized that surgical castration is not justified in postmenopausal women. In these patients, either adrenalectomy or hypophysectomy should be considered as treatment of choice. Finally, it should be mentioned that adrenalectomy and hypophysectomy are about equally effective in the control of disseminated cancer of the breast.

References

1. HUGGINS, C., HODGES, C. V.: Studies on prostatic cancer. I. The effect of castration, of estrogen, and of androgen injection on serum phosphatases in metastatic carcinoma of the prostate. Cancer Res. 1, 293 (1941).
2. LACASSAGNE, A.: Tentative pour modifier, par la progesterone ou par la testosterone, l'apparition des adenocarcinomes mammaires provoques par l'oestrone chez la souris. C. R. Soc. Biol. (Paris) 126, 385—387 (1937).
3. NATHANSON, J. T., ANDERVONT, H. B.: Effect of testosterone propionate on development and growth of mammary carcinoma in female mice. Proc. Soc. exp. Biol. (N. Y.) 40, 421—422 (1939).
4. DAO, T. L.: Hormones: Pharmacology and clinical utility in hormone related neoplasms. In: Handbook of Experimental Pharmacology, Antineoplastic and Immunosuppressive Agents. Eds.: SARTORELLI, A. C., and JOHNS, D. G. Berlin: Springer 1973 (in press).
5. BEATSON, G. T.: On the treatment of inoperable cases of carcinoma of the mamma: Suggestions for a new method of treatment with illustrative cases. Lancet 2, 104—107 (1896).
6. HUGGINS, C., BERGENSTAL, D. M.: Surgery of the adrenals. J. Amer. med. Ass. 147, 101—106 (1951).
7. LUFT, R., OLIVERCRONA, H.: Experiences with hypophysectomy in man. J. Neurosurg. 10, 301—316 (1953).
8. DAO, T. L.: Ablation therapy for hormone-dependent tumors. Ann. Rev. Med. 22, 1—18 (1972).
9. RAVDIN, R. G., LEWISON, E. F., SLACK, N. H., GARDNER, B., STATE, D., FISHER, B.: Results of a clinical trial concerning the worth of prophylactic oophorectomy for breast carcinoma. Surg Gynec. Obstet. 131, 1055—1064 (1970).
10. DAO, T. L., HUGGINS, C.: Bilateral adrenalectomy in the treatment of cancer of the breast. Arch. Surg. 71, 645—657 (1955).
11. DAO, T. L., NEMOTO, T., BROSS, I.: A controlled randomized comparative study of early and late adrenalectomy in women with advanced breast cancer. In: Prognostic Factors in Breast Cancer, pp. 177—185. Eds.: FORREST, A. P. M., and KUNKLER, P. B. Baltimore: The Williams and Wilkins Co. 1968.
12. JENSEN, E. V., DE SOMBRE, E. R., JUNGBLUT, P. W.: Estrogen receptors in hormone-responsive tissues and tumors. In: Endogenous Factors Influencing Host-Tumor Balance, pp. 15—30. Eds.: WISSLER, R. W., DAO, T. L., and WOOD, S., JR. Chicago: The University of Chicago Press 1967.
13. DAO, T. L., LIBBY, P. R.: Conjugation of steroid hormones by normal and neoplastic tissues. J. clin. Endocr. 28, 1431—1439 (1968).
14. DAO, T. L., LIBBY, P. R.: Enzymic synthesis of steroid sulfate by mammary cancer and its clinical implications. J. nat. Cancer Inst. 34, 205—210 (1971).

What Chemotherapy Should be Used in Metastatic Breast Cancer?

R. M. KELLEY

The answer to the title question is one which cannot be given with any degree of authority that is based on unequivocal scientific data. Accurate parameters for predicting the response of a given tumor to an agent or agents selected at random are not presently available and the choice of agents is still highly empirical. It cannot be otherwise until more knowledge of the cell kinetics of human breast cancer, stemming from the approaches described by Dr. MENDELSOHN, can direct us, particularly toward the timing of delivery of chemotherapy. It is obvious that the earlier an appropriate agent can be instituted and the smaller the volume of tumor cell mass, the more successful therapy is likely to be, provided that the majority of cells are in a state of active division at the time. The slow growth rate of breast cancer with the implication that the majority of cells in a given mass at any one time are likely to be in a state of temporary or permanent non-division, and thus impervious to chemical agents, renders the problem of chemotherapy much more complex than that in acute leukemia or lymphoma. Current techniques for studying human tumor cells in vitro with the incorporation of various agents in the media may help to guide the clinician in his choice of agents but at present are not applicable to the great number of patients with immediate need for treatment. Knowledge of the host's innate resistance to her tumor is implicit in successful planning of therapy, so that our choice does not interfere with, but rather enhances such resistance.

Against this background of lack of precise knowledge to dictate our therapeutic program and in view of the advanced state of disease which usually confronts the chemotherapist, it is remarkable that significant success has been achieved by the somewhat empirical application of currently available agents to a complex disease system.

Adjuvant Therapy

A logical place to attack the problem of recurrent disease is at the time of primary therapy. It is a reasonable approach to try to kill the cells which may have already metastasized to silent areas or those which may be dislodged into the systemic vascular or lymphatic circulation at the time of primary surgery, in order to decrease the recurrence rate and enhance survival by attacking implants before they are well established or theoretically free circulating tumor cells before implantation. Such an approach was assayed by the National Surgical Adjuvant Breast Project, utilizing Thio-Tepa and fluorouracil, both known to have a modicum of effectiveness against breast cancer, and a placebo. The drugs were given on the day of surgery and for two to four days thereafter. The disappointing but not surprising results of the study show no improvement in total survival at the five-year period of the treated versus control group. The study failed to take into account the concept of cell cycling and the dormant phase of many cells at the time of such limited exposure to the drugs. The effectiveness of such a program, which may hold the key to prevention of late recurrence, must await additional knowledge of cell kinetics, the potential for alteration of proliferative capacity of tumor cells to make them more vulnerable to cytotoxic agents and the development of agents potent against breast cancer which can be administered intermittently over long periods without significant toxicity to patients whose initial tumor places them at high risk for recurrence.

Choice of Patients for Chemotherapy

Faced with recurrent or initially inoperable disease, the physician has traditionally utilized some method of hormonal alteration as the first modality of therapy. This has been a practical, pragmatic course because there are some clinical guidelines to direct the choice, because toxicity is not as great as with chemotherapy and because remissions if they are induced are longer and supervision need not be so close. Since hormonal alteration is successful in only 30 to 40% of patients and ultimately fails in them, there is an enormous pool of women requring some form of palliatve chemotherapy. The earlier in the course of disease when these measures can be instituted, the more rewarding they may be. The possibility of selecting those patients with hormone-sensitive tumors by some of the approaches described by previous speakers should allow earlier institution of appropriate therapy for the remaining group. The only clinical selectivity which one may use at present is in the premenopausal woman who exhibits failure to respond to castration. Such a patient is highly unlikely to respond to further hormonal efforts and is a candidate for chemotherapy. Patients with rapidly advancing undifferentiated carcinoma, unlikely to survive long enough for a trial of hormonal therapy, should receive primary chemotherapy. Those with involvement in certain organs, particularly liver and brain and those with extensive en cuirasse, inflammatory cutaneous involvement are also unlikely to show significant response to hormonal alteration and may go directly to a chemotherapeutic program.

Despite our lack of definitive parameters for choice and timing of agents, chemotherapy is evolving as a useful tool in patients with actively progressive disease, unresponsive to hormonal therapy. Chemotherapists must be constantly aware of the narrow margin between clinical effect and toxicity so that the patient is maintained in as intact a state as possible to enjoy the palliation which may be induced. Since the agents currently utilized are all designed to attack only replicating cells, it is axiomatic that they are not specific for cancer cells, but also are active against normal cells with a rapid turn-over time, such as those of the hematopoietic system, as well as intestine and epithelial surfaces. Thus, we may deliver significant, sometimes irreversible damage to essential organs while trying to destroy tumor. Patients whose bone marrow has been compromised by extensive prior radiotherapy to osseous metastases are at great risk during vigorous chemotherapy and may not tolerate sufficient treatment to induce remission. Once the decision to use chemotherapy has been reached, dosage must be adequate to allow tumor suppression. Patients with previous adrenalectomy or hypophysectomy are extremely sensitive to toxicity and often require increased steroid coverage.

In general, the most gratifying responses to chemicals have been seen in chest wall and local soft tissue recurrences, but visceral disease and rarely, osseous involvement may also respond.

Single Drug Therapy

All of the available categories of agents have been utilized in breast cancer and responses to a wide variety of single drugs have been reported, including alkylating agents, antimetabolites, antibiotics and antimitotic compounds.

A. Fluorouracil (FU)

This anti-pyrimidine compound, an agent tailor-made to block uracil metabolism, functions by inhibiting the enzyme thymidylate synthetase. It is probably the most useful single agent in breast cancer, with a response rate reported in both randomized and non-randomized studies of 20 to 25%. Responses have been most impressive in young women who fail to respond to castration and may be maintained for a matter of several months to one or two years. Local soft tissue and hepatic metastases in particular, have demonstrated the most striking regressions, but stability of disease without either progression or regression may be maintained for long periods.

A variety of regimens for maintenance therapy are being investigated. Original recommendations were for repetitive full courses of twelve milligrams per kilo for five doses, repeated every one to two months as tolerated, inducing a fair amount of uncomfortable, but acceptable toxicity. More recently, weekly maintenance of fifteen milligrams per kilo after a loading course or even without a loading course has been utilized with good results and with much less toxicity [1]. Whether this will prove to yield as high a rate of response over as long a period as repetitive courses is not as yet clear, but there is considerable evidence that it is quite effective. The drug can be given by direct intravenous injection as an office procedure. There is accumulating information that FU is well absorbed per orum and that oral maintenance on weekly doses is feasible and effective, particularly in hepatic disease [2].

Toxicity is primarily gastrointestinal and marrow suppressive and blood counts must be monitored carefully. Stomatitis and diarrhea often follow full courses, but are rarely seen on weekly maintenance. Alopecia is observed in a small number of patients. At present, fluorouracil appears to be the drug of choice as the first chemotherapeutic agent for patients failing to respond to castration or to other modalities of hormonal therapy, particularly those who have disease limited to the liver or to the soft tissue locally and who do not have a great mass of tumor present. Osseous metastases rarely respond with objective recalcification to fluorouracil or to any other chemotherapeutic agent, but there is often times considerable subjective improvement in pain on fluorouracil.

B. Alkylating Agents

Alkylating agents react with a variety of cellular components including protein and nucleic acids, with the major action believed to result in a break in the DNA strand. Because of the relatively slow growth of breast cancer and the desirability of long term therapy, oral alkylating agents such as cyclophosphamide and chlorambucil have greater usefulness than the parenterally administered agents for systemic therapy. Remission will be seen primarily in soft tissue recurrence and slowly growing pulmonary parenchymal lesions, rarely in other sites, in about 20 to 25% of those treated for a period of a few to several months. Toxicity is primarily on the bone marrow and doses of oral preparations must be altered in accordance with frequent blood counts, particularly white cells and platelets. Cyclophosphamide has the added toxicity of alopecia and sterile hemorrhagic cystitis, but its relative platelet sparing effect enhances its usefulness. Combination with prednisone often complements the effectiveness of oral alkylating agents and allows the administration of larger doses for longer periods by its supportive bone marrow effect.

A particular indication for alkylating agents is in the local control of pleural effusions when they are due to involvement of the serosal surface with small tumor implants. Both triethylene thiophosphoramide (Thio-Tepa) and nitrogen mustard are effective in controlling effusions in patients whose only evidence of recurrence is the effusion or in those where recurrent effusion is the most symptomatic manifestation of widespread disease under therapy with other measures. It may be necessary to instill them two or three times in any given effusion before a therapeutic effect is achieved or to introduce them after tube thoracotomy drainage to allow adherence of pleural surfaces prior to instillation of agent. In patients receiving systemic chemotherapy in addition to the local instillation, blood counts must be watched carefully because there is some systemic absorption across the pleural surface.

C. Folic Acid Antagonist — Methotrexate

One of the most important developments of the past few years in chemotherapy has been the emergence of methotrexate as an agent with a potential far beyond that originally demonstrated by Dr. FARBER in acute childhood leukemia. Breast cancer is one of several solid tumors in which this agent has been occasionally effective. It works by blocking the conversion of folic acid to tetrahydrofolic acid, an essential step in the building of nucleoprotein. Approximately 15 to 20% of patients with breast cancer will respond for a few months, either to daily divided oral doses of 2.5—5.0 mg q.d. or to intravenous injections of 0.4—0.6 mg/kg twice weekly.

Toxicity may be considerable to the bone marrow and the GI tract and methotrexate is contraindicated in patients with impaired renal function because of its excretion via the kidneys.

D. Vinca Alkaloids

Both vinblastine and vincristine have demonstrated limited ability to induce regressions in breast cancer, particularly local involvement, occasionally in cases where other agents have not been effective. Velban is a relatively safe drug with some marrow toxicity while vincristine is marrow sparing, but neurotoxic. Their usefulness is somewhat limited by the need for weekly intravenous injections and by intense perivascular irritation, if leaked into the surrounding tissues.

E. Multiple Drug Therapy

It is evident from the discussion so far, that the usefulness of chemotherapeutic agents singly in extensive disease is rather modest in terms of percentage, duration and site of responsiveness and that a more effective approach is necessary, if possible, with the agents presently available. The sequential use of the agents, although sometimes of real benefit, may be limited by marrow exhaustion and by inexorably advancing disease with depletion of the patient.

The concept of total kill of cancer cells by combination therapy so promising in acute childhood leukemia is not so easily applied to solid tumors for reasons previously mentioned. Nevertheless, an attempt to attain a summation of therapeutic effect, a delay in development of drug resistance, and possible diminution in toxicity by using lower doses of agents at different sites of intracellular vulnerability to achieve a more effective metabolic blockade of cell growth is very appealing in breast cancer. Fear of intolerable toxicity from combined chemotherapy has proved less formidable than anticipated and with extreme caution in dosage and frequency of administration, additive toxicity has been a controllable problem, in patients not too nutritionally depleted or subjected to extensive prior chemotherapy or radiotherapy.

GREENSPAN [3] for several years has utilized a combination of Thio-Tepa or other alkylating agents with methotrexate with and without fluorouracil in varying combinations, with prednisone, testosterone and B-12 as supplements to protect the bone marrow and has recorded a 50 to 60% response rate, particularly in patients with hepatic and pulmonary metastases and skin involvement. Such responses have been maintained usually for only a few months but a small percentage of cases have responded for up to two years.

TALLEY et al. [4] have reported results of a Phase I evaluation of a triple drug combination of cyclophosphamide, vincristine and fluorouracil and recorded a higher incidence of response than would have been anticipated with any single agent.

The most recent effort at combined therapy, and one receiving wide therapeutic trial at present, is the so-called Cooper Regimen [5], a five-drug program, initially reported as giving a 90% response rate in women with disease in sites not usually responding favorably, such as intracranial, hepatic and inflammatory skin involvement. This program (Table) consists of daily oral cyclophosphamide and prednisone and weekly intravenous doses of fluorouracil, methotrexate and vincristine for eight

Table. Cooper regimen [5]

First 10—12 wks		
5-Fluorouracil (5-FU)	12 mg/kg	I.V. weekly
Methotrexate (MTX)	0.6 mg/kg	I.V. weekly
Vincristine (VCR)	0.35 µg/kg (4—6 wks only)	I.V. weekly
Prednisone (PRED.)	0.75 mg/kg daily p.o. for 2 wks, then declining doses to 5 mg maintenance	
Cyclophosphamide (CYT.)	2 mg/kg	daily p.o.
Maintenance as tolerated		

to twelve weeks, if possible, with maintenance at more widely spaced intervals and
with dosages varying depending upon marrow reserve and toxic effects. Such a program can be carried out on an outpatient basis, with many patients developing little
or no symptomatic toxicity except for alopecia, which is total in nearly all cases.
Marked marrow depression has been seen, however, after just one cycle of therapy in
patients whose marrow is in jeopardy due to disease or previous therapy and over-
whelming sepsis has occurred in these circumstances. Regressions of hepatic, intracranial and en cuirasse skin involvement have been impressive in several cases and
have been maintained for several months to over one year. Many such regressions,
however, have been disappointingly brief. This is not a drug schedule to be offered
to all hormone-resistant cases and patients must be carefully chosen who are in
relatively good condition despite the inroads of their disease and whose disease cannot
be expected to respond to other, simpler approaches. Knowledge of the intrinsic
toxicity of each drug is implicit in multi-agent management so that the program can
be altered week by week as necessary. Schedules such as these should be initiated and
maintained only with the advice of the trained oncologist, although once instituted
the drugs can be administered by the primary physician. Vigorous treatment of inter-
current infection may be necessary on such a schedule.

The contribution of each drug individually to the observed responses is difficult
to evaluate and it may be that all five drugs are not necessary or that a different
schedule of the same drugs may yield a higher percentage of remissions. Many studies
of various combinations of the basic drugs and their timing are currently under study
by the national cooperative groups, the National Cancer Institute group and individual investigators. Preliminary reports suggest that all five drugs may not be
necessary and that combinations omitting one or two of the drugs may be equally
effective, with less toxicity, more sustained maintenance possibilities and greater
economy. The five-drug program is expensive. As new drugs are demonstrated to
have efficacy against breast cancer they will undoubtedly be incorporated in these
regimens for trial.

Despite all of these advances, the oncologist faced with a succession of patients
with disseminated breast cancer is constantly aware that he is delivering too little too
late, that he may be tampering with the hosts' innate immune defenses by introducing
the right drugs at the wrong times or the wrong drugs at all times, that his best efforts
must remain tangential to the problem until the fruition at the clinical level of the
results of sophisticated laboratory studies of enzymatic and immune systems, of cell
kinetics and cellular control mechanisms, of drug pharmacology and interactions of
drugs, of drugs with greater anti-tumor activity, of mechanisms of development of
drug resistance, et cetera. The efforts of the basic scientists involved in these approaches to solid tumors will render the clinical answer to the title question quite
different in five to ten years, I believe. Perhaps in a few more years we may obviate
entirely the need to discuss therapy for late breast cancer because adequate methods
of early detection and appropriate primary and adjuvant therapy may so dilute the
problem.

References

1. HORTON, J., OLSON, K. B., SULLIVAN, J., REILLY, C., SHNIDER, B.: Eastern Coop. Oncology
   Group. 5-Fluorouracil in cancer: An improved regimen. Ann. intern. Med. 73, 897—900
   (1970).

2. IRWIN, L. E., PUGH, R. P., BRAUNWALD, J.: Western Coop. Cancer Chemotherapy Group. 5-Fluorouracil given once weekly: Comparison of I. V. and oral administration. Amer. Soc. clin. Oncol., Inc. Abstract 32 (1971).
3. GREENSPAN, E. M.: Combination cytotoxic chemotherapy in advanced disseminated breast carcinoma. J. Mt Sinai Hosp. 33, 1—27 (1966).
4. TUCKER, W. G., TALLEY, R. W., BROWNLEE, R. W., BURROWS, J. H., STOTT, P. B., MOOR-HEAD, E. L., SAN DIEGO, E. L.: Preliminary trials with combination chemotherapy of cyclo-phosphamide, vincristine and 5-fluorouracil (CON-FU). Cancer Chemother. Abstr. 52, 5 (1968).
5. COOPER, R. G.: Combination chemotherapy in hormone resistant breast cancer. Proc. Amer. Ass. Cancer Res. 10, 15 (1969).

Epilogue

P. P. Carbone

Cancer Teaching Symposium on Breast Cancer: A Challenging Problem

As my first duty on behalf of the other participants and myself, I must recognize and thank our wonderful hosts Drs. Griem, Wissler, Ultmann and Jensen for the excellent accommodations and for a most stimulating conference for us the participants as well as the listeners. Two years ago for the Lymphoma-Leukemia Conference my impressions of the results of these conferences were so positive that I accepted immediately the invitation to attend this meeting on breast cancer. I hope the organizers find an appropriate subject in my field for the next conference. Thanks again.

I am supposed to summarize the proceedings of the entire conference. Dr. John Ultmann in his highly energetic way suggested that I either do a complete task of summarizing 11 hours of lectures in 20 minutes or disregard what has been said and give an entirely different lecture. As a compromise, I will try to do some of both, adding some of my ideas on breast cancer.

The conference had as its main theme the idea that research in epidemiology, mammary tumor cell biology, and clinical investigation will lead to better ways of prevention, detection and treatment (Fig. 1).

One must collect baseline information and select those factors that are controllable and determine control measures for appropriate populations (Fig. 2). These ideas must be tested and confirmed by clinical trials, so that the best agents and modalities can be applied in the appropriate groups of patients. Breast cancer can be analyzed on the basis of its biologic, clinical, and histologic features, namely non-invasive, local disease with low metastatic potential, local disease with high metastatic potential, regional disease, spread to local nodes and tissues, and metastatic. As part of any program, the results must be tabulated, evaluated, and disseminated.

The conference started with the expression of optimism by Dean Leon Jacobson who inferred that much progress against breast cancer had been achieved in the last 20 years. As with most pronouncements by deans these days, his statement did not go unchallenged, because the next two speakers stressed the lack of progress noting that the mortality had not changed appreciably in the last 60 years. Dr. Letton offered the American Cancer Society's program of improving the cure rate in human breast cancer by providing for early detection. Data from the HIP study in New York where random allocation of patients to routine mammography and physical examination or no followup except as indicated, provide important evidence to indicate

that routine screening significantly decreases the overall mortality by 50% [1].
Dr. LETTON also stressed rehabilitation of the breast cancer patient as an important
goal.

Dr. M. SHIMKIN very aptly summarized the epidemiology of breast cancer. He
noted the relatively narrow range of incidence rates (about 6-fold from the lowest to
the highest), in contrast to lung or esophageal cancer or hepatic cancer where the rates

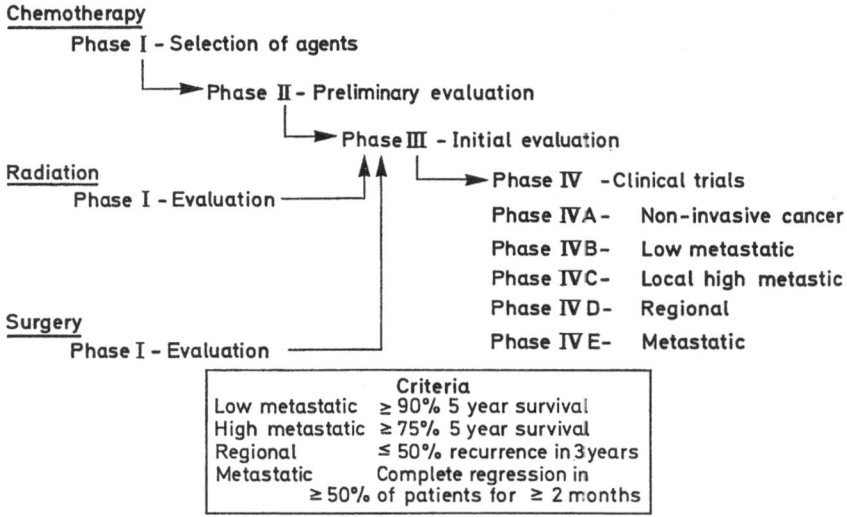

Fig. 1. Breast cancer program: NCI Breast Cancer task force flow diagram

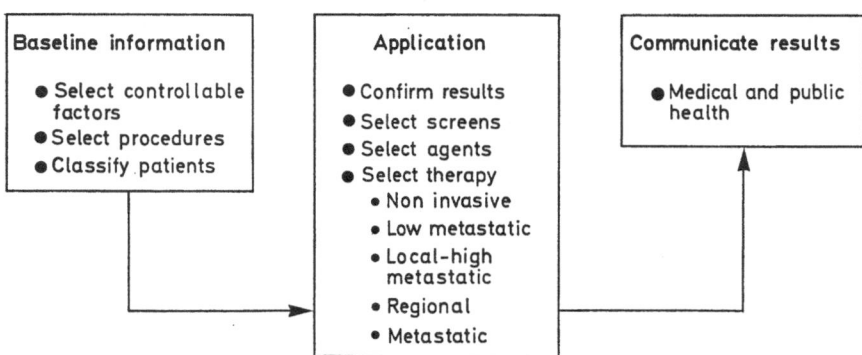

Fig. 2. Breast cancer program: NCI Breast Cancer task force flow diagram

might vary 100-fold. He implied that this probably precluded external environmental
factors in etiology. However, a simple physical fact may help explain the difference
in incidence between American and Japanese women. Some of my traveling friends
and others have noted the relatively small breasts of Japanese women as compared to
Americans. Besides the geographical differences, he stressed that only a history of one
breast cancer or a history of other breast conditions increased the risk of breast cancer

by more than 2-fold. Steroid discriminants, he described as peripheral and recommended more attention to measurement of binding proteins.

Recently, another factor has been described as related to susceptibility to viral disease. This applies to linked susceptibility to virus disease and antigen recognization in mice that has been related to genetic factors in mice and to HL-A types in man [2, 3]. TERASAKI has described a low gene frequency in Japanese of HL-A 1 that is higher in Americans and in breast cancer patients [4].

Dr. N. SARKAR reported on the characteristics of the mouse mammary tumor virus and suggested a candidate virus for man. This brings up the added concern of trying to prevent reinduction of second breast cancers, because even if we can detect and treat early breast cancer, the incidence of a second breast cancer in the opposite breast will continue to rise unless thwarted by effective virus inhibition.

Dr. M. LIPSETT despaired about discussing hormonal carcinogenesis, stressing that even in the mouse, a well-understood system, we still did not have a unified concept to explain oncogenesis. He reviewed the various exogenous factors that might influence hormonal metabolism such as thyroid status, obesity, and fat in diet. He described the difficulties of relating urine steroid levels or prolactin levels to breast cancer suspectibility but was optimistic in measuring estrone sulfate by a sensitive radioimmunoassay technique. Estrone sulfate has a long half-life and is a reflection of estrogen production in man.

Dr. B. J. KENNEDY presented a very graphic clinical lecture on the biology of human breast cancer. He stressed the role of early detection in decreasing the mortality of cancer by picking up small lesions without lymph node enlargement. He described recent studies by CUTLER and TAYLOR in establishing a possible staging scheme for patients with advanced disease. "Dire prognosis sites" included the liver, brain, peritoneum, and spinal cord with a 6-month median survival time (MST). Other single sites were less serious, resulting in a MST of 10 months [5].

Dr. R. EGAN described his studies with x-ray mammography introduced since the 1960's. His studies have indicated a high degree (90%) of accuracy in picking up lesions in the breast. Other studies have reported that palpation as well as mammography are important concomitant procedures that should be used. He described the indications for routine mammography as previous breast disease, cancer in the opposite breast, and family history of breast cancer. At present no other technique, thermography, isotopic scanning, or ultrasound, offers any advantages over mammography and palpation. Assuming that Dr. EGAN would pick up small lesions of 1 or 2 mm^3, these still contain 10^6 cells, or at least 15 doublings of tumor cells. The role of calcification in the tumor remains unexplained and intriguing.

Dr. D. SCARPELLI presented new data on the use of histochemistry and electron microscopy in breast cancer. He stressed the need to identify the cell of origin. However, Dr. ULTMANN raised the question about the need to identify subtypes, Table [6]. Eighty % of tumors are ductal carcinomas. This situation is reminiscent of the state of affairs in Hodgkin's disease with the old Jackson-Parker classification and before the Rye classification. We must develop more refined tools to evaluate the classification.

Dr. E. JENSEN described his elegant studies in the development of a biochemical predictor of response to hormonal ablation or treatment. An understanding of hormone action and newer techniques of measurement have allowed the development of a highly predictive test. He measures the binding protein of estrogen, radiolabeled, and the ability to suppress its binding by specific inhibitors *in vitro*. He has shown that 13/17 patients with the binding protein responded and only 1/32 responded who did not have the binding protein. He reported recent results from Germany confirming these studies. It would appear that it might be possible to develop a potent inhibitor that might replace ablative surgery and one such drug, nafoxidine, is in clinical test in Europe [7].

Table. Classification of breast cancer

AFIP Fascicle
  I. Non infiltrating duct carcinoma
    (1) Papillary (cribriform)
    (2) Solid (comedo)
  II. Infiltrating duct carcinoma
    (1) Scirrhous   80%
    (2) Comedo   5%
    (3) Medullary 5%
    (4) Papillary   1.5%
    (5) Colloid   0.2%
  III. Paget's disease of the nipple
  IV. Non-infiltrating lobular carcinoma
   V. Infiltrating lobular carcinoma 5%
  VI. Rare carcinomas
    (1) Sweat gland (apocrine)
    (2) Adenoid cystic
    (3) Tubular
    (4) Inflammatory
    (5) Metaplastic lesions
       (a) cartilage
       (b) spindle
       (c) squamous

Improving the host's inherent immunity has become the hope of the immunologists as the approach to treatment. Dr. G. HEPPNER has shown elegantly in the mouse system how drug induced immune suppression might be used to inhibit blocking antibody and allow cellular immunity to do its duty. More recently, Dr. E. HERSH [8] and Dr. B. LEVENTHAL [9] have shown that drug treatment of leukemia may, in fact, improve immunity to nonspecific antigen as well as to leukemia cells. One test that Dr. HEPPNER did not mention was skin testing with cell membranes, a procedure found to be useful in Burkitt's tumor and leukemia [10].

Dr. M. MENDELSOHN described the important implications of tumor cell kinetics for therapists and biologists but expressed pessimism because of the relatively difficult technique to measure the necessary components of cell cycle time, growth fraction, and the stem cell compartment. Concern was expressed over our inability to study the stem cell compartment. Yet, there are probably two *in vitro* assays that may measure clonigenic cells. Dr. BERGSAGEL and his group have been able to grow murine and human plasma cells *in vitro* [11], and several authors including ourselves report growth of marrow cells in culture. It may be a problem that may need to be studied more directly such as with the functional assay like clone formation. From experimental studies the kinetics vary with the size of the tumor and change after treatment. One possible approach would be to develop a marker of tumor cell numbers that can be used like alpha feto protein and human chorionic gonadotrophin to follow tumor cell mass.

Dr. M. MYERS presented data of the End Results Section of NCI with over 70,000 cases of breast cancer. The overall incidence rates 74/100,000 seems to be leveling off. Mortality has not changed in the last 30 years. For localized disease, regional disease, and all stages the mortality has stabilized at the 1955 figures. Of most importance was the finding that statistical definition of cure rates, i. e. the mortality rate equal to that of the normal population, has not been achieved at any time interval up to 20 years after diagnosis.

Dr. W. RIDER presented a plea for more localized therapy of breast cancer by x-ray therapy and possibly for primary treatment with these modalities. He ennumerated several reasons, radical mastectomy may be on the wane. Dr. W. BURDETTE emphasized the need to concentrate on treatment of patients with disseminated disease, that is 60% of patients. One of the difficulties in combining modalities is the large number of possible combinations of modalities. He suggested two alternatives, 1. earlier diagnosis and conservative use of radical mastectomy, and 2. development of more effective systemic treatment.

Dr. R. NISSEN-MEYER described four prospective randomized clinical trials in Scandinavia. The use of primary radiation castration in premenopausal women, characterized as having a low risk of recurrences, and in postmenopausal women resulted in a significant prolongation of disease free period but not of survival. A comparison of surgical versus radiation castration was carried out in pre-menopausal women with high risk of recurrence and indicated a more effective result with radiation castration. The fourth study employing postoperative cyclophosphamide decreased the recurrences and improved survival.

The problem of treatment of systemic disease was discussed by Drs. T. DAO and R. KELLEY. Dr. DAO described the results of hormonal manipulation. The use of exogenous hormones, despite attempts at biochemical manipulation of the molecule, results in a response rate to androgens and estrogens of about 20%. Dr. DAO reported the improved value of adrenalectomy early in the course of relapse rather than late. Of great interest was the report of steroid sulfate conjugation measurements indicating that there are populations of tumor cells existing that have the enzyme. Response to adrenalectomy correlated highly with a high DHEA/17B ratio for sulfation.

Dr. KELLEY mentioned the traditional role of the chemotherapist as the final practitioner. She hoped that this role will change with new knowledge of cell kinetics and *in vitro* measurements of sensitivity. She recommended early use of adjuvant chemotherapy following operative treatment. The general trend is to use hormonal alteration, then chemotherapy. Patients with premenopausal castration failure, tumor in the liver or brain, or with inflammatory carcinoma are candidates for early chemotherapy. Gratifying responses occur with chemotherapy even with visceral disease. Early reports of combination chemotherapy are hopeful.

Thus, the treatment of breast cancer will depend on the optimal use of radiation therapy, chemotherapy including immunotherapy, and endocrine therapy and surgery

(Fig. 3). We must develop to its maximum each of these modalities through research, and test them in combinations where necessary. These trials must be specific for subgroups of breast cancer patients. The NCI Breast Cancer Task Force has defined these into five groups: non-invasive cancer, local cancer with low metastatic potential, local disease with high potential of spread, regional metastasis, and distant metastatic disease. We must design our treatment programs for specific classes of patients. As shown in Fig. 3, the Breast Cancer Task Force has set criteria of success for each sub-

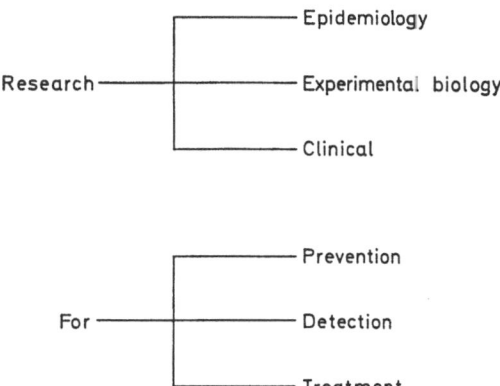

Fig. 3. Breast cancer program: NCI Breast Cancer task force flow diagram

group and will aim to improve on these. The classification of patients depends on parameters related to clinical stage and to histologic features, such as nuclear grade, blood vessel invasion, and node status. Hopefully, we can define the absolute risk of recurrence for specific patients and apply treatment modalities other than surgery earlier in the natural course. With more rational treatment and earlier diagnosis, we can hope that fewer women will die of breast cancer, although we may not be able to prevent the disease. Ultimately, our goal will be to prevent induction or reverse the malignant process.

Acknowledgements

I want to thank Dr. N. BERLIN, Chairman, NCI Breast Cancer Task Force, and Dr. A. S. KETCHAM for permission to refer to the activities of the Breast Cancer Task Force and the use of materials (Figs. 1, 2, 3).

References

1. VENET, L., STRAX, P., VENET, W., SHAPIRO, S.: Adequacies and inadequacies of breast examination by physicians in mass screening. Cancer (Philad.) 28, 1546—1551 (1971).
2. LILLY, F., BOYSE, E. A., OLD, L. J.: Genetic basis of susceptibility to viral leukemogenesis. Lancet 1964 II, 1207—1209.
3. McDEVITT, H. D., BODMER, W. F.: Histocompatibility antigens, immune responsiveness and susceptibility to disease. Amer. J. Med. 52, 1—8 (1972).
4. TERASAKI, P.: Unpublished data.

5. CUTLER, S. J., ASIRE, A. J., TAYLOR, S. G.: Classification of patients with disseminated cancer of the breast. Cancer (Philad.) 24, 861—869 (1969).
6. McDEVITT, R. W., STEWART, F. W., BERG, J. W.: Tumors of the Breast. In: Atlas of Tumor Pathology, second series, fascicle 2. Washington, D. C.: Armed Forces Institute of Pathology 1968.
7. TAGNON, H.: Personal communication.
8. CHEEMA, A. R., HERSH, E. M.: Patient survival after chemotherapy and its relationship to in vitro lymphocyte blastogenesis. Cancer (Philad.) 28, 851—856 (1971).
9. HALTERMAN, R. H., LEVENTHAL, B. G.: Enhanced immune response to leukemia. Lancet 1971 II, 704—705.
10. BLUMING, A. Z., ZIEGLER, J. L., FASS, L., HERBEN, R. E.: Delayed cutaneous sensitivity reactions to autologous Burkitt lymphoma protein extract. Clin. exp. Immun. 9, 713 (1971).
11. OGAWA, M., BERGSAGEL, D. E., McCULLOCH, E. A.: Chemotherapy of mouse myeloma: Quantitative cell cultures predictive of response in vivo. Blood 41, 7—15 (1973).

Recent Results
in Cancer Research

Sponsored by the Swiss League against Cancer
Editor in chief: P. Rentchnick, Geneva

In Production

In Preparation

     Prices are subject to change without notice.

---

* Distribution rights for U. K., Commonwealth and the Traditional British Market (excluding Canada): W. Heinemann, Medical Books Ltd., London.